FREEZE!

HOW YOU CAN
HELP PREVENT
NUCLEAR WAR

BY SENATOR
EDWARD M. KENNEDY
AND SENATOR
MARK O. HATFIELD

FOREWORD BY
W. AVERELL HARRIMAN

BANTAM
Toronto • New York

D0210055

FREEZE!
HOW YOU CAN HELP PREVENT NUCLEAR WAR

A Bantam Book / April 1982

All Rights Reserved

ISBN 0-553-14077-9

Published simultaneously in the United States and Canada

PRINTED IN THE UNITED STATES OF AMERICA

0 9 8 7 6 5 4 3 2 1

To all the members of
the nuclear freeze movement, who
have awakened the conscience
of our country and who are proving
anew that individuals truly
can make a difference.

ACKNOWLEDGMENTS

The preparation of this manuscript required the hard work, dedication and commitment of many superbly talented people. We are pleased to have had many such people give unstintingly of their time and energies to this project.

We are especially grateful to Carey Parker and Robert Shrum for the preparation and compilation of much of the material in this book. Their expertise, enthusiasm, patience and meticulous attention to detail are clearly reflected in the quality of this product.

Lawrence Horowitz, Jan Kalicki, Rick Rolf, and Matthew Murray also made major contributions in preparing this book, in developing the Kennedy-Hatfield Nuclear Freeze Resolution itself and in forging a coalition of support for it.

We feel fortunate to have been able to test our ideas and share our drafts with some of the most knowledgeable experts in the field, including Jonathan Medalia, Christopher Paine, Jeffrey Porro, Peter Sharfman, John Steinbruner, Jeremy Stone and Paul Warnke.

The preparation of this manuscript in a relatively brief period of time would not have been possible without the extraordinary work of Tom Getman, Matthew State, Ellen Blaisdell, Barbara Cobb, Nancy Dalton, Ann Fielder, Alice Gallasch, Eather Higginbotham, Terry Hitchins, Annie Jones, Mark Kramer, Constance Lambert, Tom Maginnis, Patricia McHugh, Sarah Milam, Bruce Morgan, John Packs, Laverne Walker, Sandra Walker, Joanne Yancey, and many others.

Finally we want to thank the members of the national nuclear weapons freeze movement, who gave us the inspiration for this book and who have given their country a new chance to stop the nuclear arms race.

CONTENTS

FOREWORD

Twenty-six years ago, to the very day that I compose this Foreword, President Eisenhower wrote of the age of nuclear weapons:

> . . . the true security problem of the day . . . is not merely man against man or nation against nation. It is man against war. . . . When we get to the point, as one day we will, that both sides know that in any outbreak of general hostilities, regardless of the element of surprise, destruction will be both reciprocal and complete, possibly we will have sense enough to meet at the conference table with the understanding that the era of armaments has ended and the human race must conform its actions to this truth or die.

Twenty-six years ago, neither the United States nor the Soviet Union had deployed a single strategic intercontinental missile. Today, our nations together have deployed thousands of strategic missiles carrying many more thousands of even larger nuclear warheads. These are not ponderous bombers that we can recall. Flying at more than ten thousand miles an hour, they are irrevocable weapons with minutes for flight and seconds for decision.

Twenty-six years ago, three nations had set off nuclear explosions. Today, that number is six, and ten more nations could join them by the end of this decade.

Twenty-six years ago, the memory of global conflict was

fresh in the minds of all; we were resolved that war should never come again because nations feared to negotiate or negotiated from fear. Today, two generations have grown up in the United States and the Soviet Union, knowing nothing of the crucible and the calvary of that gradually dimming conflagration.

Twenty-six years ago, the leaders and scientists who determined the choices about nuclear weapons were the men who had constructed them and felt the flash of heat upon their faces from explosions set off a score of miles away. Today, these collective memories are fading, and too few have any idea of the scale of force the United States and the Soviet Union have assembled and the awesome power man now holds within his hands.

Nuclear war would be an unparalleled catastrophe. It is the ultimate challenge to American security for it threatens our very survival. No one used to the freedom and liberty of America can comprehend a society shattered; a once-great nation prey to any other caring to walk in our debris. For the Soviet Union, which I saw undergo the trauma of losing twenty million citizens in four years, all-out nuclear war could bring one hundred and twenty million dead in four days. For the rest of this world, as this book so vividly details, nuclear war could threaten the very existence of life itself.

Too many today are seriously considering the idea of limited nuclear war. This idea is not the harmless dreaming of madmen locked in a cage. It is determining the weapons that are built and the strategies for their use, and it is encouraging the nuclear choice by telling all nations that nuclear weapons are just another instrument of power. I refuse to believe that our humanity and nobility and wisdom have so diminished that we would hand over our future to those who say that with nuclear weapons there can be a "surgical" nuclear strike, or that human restraint will still prevail with millions dead after a so-called "limited" nuclear attack.

Too many today are seriously considering the idea of civil defense as the answer to the threat of nuclear war. The truth, to paraphrase Joe Louis, is that in a nuclear war you can run, but you cannot hide. Effective civil defense in a nuclear war is utterly impractical. I refuse to believe that our common sense has so diminished that we would hand over our future to those who say that with civil defense the economies of the United States and the Soviet Union would recover in two to four years.

Nuclear weapons exist for one purpose only—to deter nuclear war. Once used, they will consume the destroyer as well as the destroyed.

It is urgent, therefore, that we act now, and that is the message of this book and the reason behind a nuclear freeze. There are fifty thousand nuclear warheads in the world today, and this number is growing. Weapons are about to be deployed that would compel one side to strike first in a crisis. Other weapons are about to be deployed that will be difficult to verify with confidence and thus extremely difficult to restrain.

Potential nuclear powers are waiting in the wings. And nuclear terrorism presents the possibility of no deterrence at all; a nuclear bomb could be exploded on an American city and we might not know from where it came. It is the ultimate bad dream, for it is the one which we may soon discover is not a dream but a nightmare come true.

It is urgent that we act now to take advantage of the window of opportunity still open for us before these developments and other come to pass, for, if the history of man's attempts to control nuclear arms has taught us anything, it is that opportunities lost in time become opportunities lost forever.

We must begin serious negotiations with the Soviet Union and agree to mutual restraint while we negotiate. The word "serious" is vital, for some in both nations will counsel proposals designed to be rejected by the other side—useful as an excuse for doing nothing.

It is folly to assume that there is any course other than negotiated control of nuclear arms, and it is foolhardy to believe that we can afford to wait. In the nuclear age, such controls offer the only way to limit the forces arrayed against us. Without such controls, we will be able to add more to our forces, but so will the Soviets be able to add more to theirs. This will leave them free to field every one of their new generation of missiles, and free to add thousands of additional warheads. I believe that it would be a curious as well as a dangerous program of national security that would permit the

Soviet Union to target an unlimited number of hydrogen warheads against our country.

It is compounded folly to assume that better control of nuclear arms can result from a race to nuclear superiority. We understand now—all too clearly—how the failure to limit multiple independently-targetable warheads ten years ago has come back to haunt the very missiles they were designed to enhance. My reading of the Soviet experience—and I have met with every Soviet leader from Stalin to Brezhnev—indicates that Moscow will make whatever sacrifice it takes to remain equal—as we will too. The conclusion will not be superiority; the end will be an arms race without end.

Nuclear stability comes when neither side feels inferior, and this is the true margin of safety.

There is in the Soviet Union a spectrum of opinion in its ruling group, ranging from hardliners to those who have a more reasonable attitude and who are concerned with the development of the Soviet Union for the benefit of its people. There will be no security for our nation if a new generation of Soviet leaders comes to power in the midst of an unconstrained arms race where the only hope we have is that reason will prevail over uncertainty, suspicion, and fear.

I am convinced that Soviet leaders, young and old, desire serious negotiations. Such negotiations will not be easy, for these talks will be—as they have always been—hard-headed exercises to improve the national security of both countries. They will not signal our approval of other Soviet actions, such as martial law in Poland. Their object, despite the irreconcilable ideologies of our two nations, simply is the common goal that nuclear weapons have made the prevention of nuclear war a necessity. Somehow, both our nations must fashion, in the words of President Kennedy, "a middle ground between the peace of the grave and the security of the slave."

Nothing can paralyze this search for security and safety more surely than the belief of either nation that the other is superior in nuclear weapons. Today, the strategic nuclear forces of the United States and the Soviet Union are equivalent in strength. The Soviets have more missiles and bombers combined; our missiles and bombers can deliver more weapons. More of the Soviet deterrent force is carried on land-based missiles; more of ours is carried aboard long-range bombers and missile-firing submarines.

The myth of Soviet superiority not only paralyzes, but it reflects fear, a fear unworthy of this most confident of nations. It strains credulity as well, for, even after the most succesful Soviet surprise attack seriously contemplated, we could respond with some four to five thousand nuclear weapons. This myth demoralizes our friends, but, worst of all, it sets the stage for deadly and avoidable miscalculation by telling our opponents we are weak when in fact we are not.

The purpose of this book is to engage Americans in the choice about their future. This engagement has already begun spontaneously in hundreds of town meetings across this country, and it is spreading rapidly.

This engagement gives me confidence. Twice before, the American people have been involved in the control of nuclear arms, and twice before there has been progress. Twenty years ago, popular concern over nuclear war and fallout from nuclear testing led to the signing of the Limited Test Ban Treaty which forbade all nuclear tests by the superpowers except those conducted underground. Ten years ago, the national debate over the deployment of anti-ballistic missiles led to the signing of the SALT I Anti-Ballistic Missile Treaty which prevented a race in expensive and unworkable defensive systems, as well as a race in offensive missiles to overcome them.

Now is the time for Americans to learn about nuclear weapons: about the dangers they pose and what can be done. It is also the time to speak out. This volume addresses both these requirements in straightforward and eloquent terms.

The issues presented by nuclear arms are not partisan. Correctly, one of the authors of this book, Senator Kennedy, is a Democrat and the other, Senator Hatfield, is a Republican. Such bi-partisan statesmanship is necessary, for in the face of this issue we are all Americans, and the future of America is inextricably linked with the future of arms control. Even more fundamentally, we are all human beings, seeking to preserve a planet and its vital seed of life.

This goal will require a collective expression of human will, and it will require our country's leadership. No other nation has our power and unique capabilities. No other nation can provide the leadership that peace demands. That leadership will be the finest expression of America's dream. We dare not fail.

Civilization has existed for perhaps ten thousand years. In our short time on earth, we are given a choice about the kind of world we leave behind. With nuclear weapons in our custody, those who inhabit the earth today carry a heavy obligation. There will be no historian to record that we failed in our watch.

W. Averell Harriman
Washington, D. C.
April 12, 1982

INTRODUCTION

On March 10, 1982, we introduced a congressional resolution calling for a mutual and verifiable nuclear weapons freeze between the United States and the Soviet Union, followed by negotiations for major reductions in nuclear arsenals. The resolution was sponsored in the House of Representatives by Edward J. Markey and Silvio O. Conte of Massachusetts, and Jonathan B. Bingham of New York. At this writing, it has the support of more than 190 members of Congress. Already, the Kennedy-Hatfield resolution has helped to focus the nation's attention on the critical issues of nuclear arms control and nuclear war. But in its truest sense, the resolution is the result of a grassroots movement across America.

At the press conference when the resolution was announced, we stood with representatives of the freeze movement, with religious leaders, and with arms control experts who perceive the urgency of a new approach to stop the accelerating nuclear arms race. The Kennedy-Hatfield resolution has been endorsed by a wide range of individuals and organizations, not all of them directly involved in the nuclear issue. Members of the Wilderness Society understand, for example, that their hopes and purposes can never be achieved in a world transformed into a nuclear wilderness. The President of the National Organization for Women understands that this is a central issue for all human beings. Citizen support for a nuclear freeze has mounted across the country. Hundreds of town meetings have passed freeze resolutions; city councils and state legislatures have approved similar resolutions; a statewide referendum will be on the ballot this November in California and grassroots efforts are under way to put it on the ballot in other states.

The Kennedy-Hatfield resolution is the only measure be-

fore the Congress which has the endorsement of the National
Nuclear Weapons Freeze Campaign. Its wording parallels
that of the Massachusetts and California nuclear freeze initiatives. The resolution is a clear and compelling call which
any citizen can read and which every citizen can answer. The
text is understandable and unequivocal:

> Whereas the greatest challenge facing the earth is
> to prevent the occurrence of nuclear war by acci-
> dent or design;
> Whereas the nuclear arms race is dangerously in-
> creasing the risk of a holocaust that would be hu-
> manity's final war; and
> Whereas a freeze followed by reductions in nu-
> clear warheads, missiles, and other delivery systems
> is needed to halt the nuclear arms race and to
> reduce the risk of nuclear war;
> Resolved by the Senate and the House of
> Representatives of the United States of America in
> Congress assembled,
> 1. As an immediate strategic arms control objec-
> tive, the United States and the Soviet Union
> should:
> (a) pursue a complete halt to the nuclear arms
> race;
> (b) decide when and how to achieve a mutual
> and verifiable freeze on the testing, production, and
> further deployment of nuclear warheads, missiles,
> and other delivery systems; and
> (c) give special attention to destabilizing weap-
> ons whose deployment would make such a freeze
> more difficult to achieve.
> 2. Proceeding from this freeze, the United States
> and the Soviet Union should pursue major, mutual,
> and verifiable reductions in nuclear warheads, mis-
> siles, and other delivery systems, through annual
> percentages or equally effective means, in a manner
> that enhances stability.

Both of us have been involved in the struggle for arms
control for all of our public lives. We have discussed it with
American and Soviet Presidents and fought for it on the
Senate floor. The Kennedy-Hatfield resolution is the latest

step in that continuing effort. We offer this book not only as
a case for the nuclear freeze, but as a manual for citizen involvement in the struggle. The book discusses the risks and
consequences of nuclear war, the limited successes and past
failures of arms control, and the strategy for achieving a nuclear freeze. Chapter Nine answers the fifty most important
questions about a freeze, and Chapter Ten offers specific suggestions for citizen action. In this book, you can find out
what will happen to your own city or town in the event of a
nuclear war, and you will learn what you can do to help prevent that war from happening. Much of what you read in
these pages is horrifying, but much of it is hopeful as well.
The dangers are great, but the opportunities for peaceful
progress are equally great. We believe this book can make at
least a small contribution to that progress.

Edward M. Kennedy
Mark O. Hatfield
Washington, D. C.
April 12, 1982

1

THE FIRST
NUCLEAR WAR

"Japan, after all, not only survived but flourished after the nuclear attack."

—Eugene Rostow
Director, U.S. Arms Control and
Disarmament Agency

The notion that nuclear war is survivable and winnable, in any meaningful sense, has become increasingly and dangerously fashionable among a certain school of strategic analysts as well as among some officials of both the Reagan and Carter administrations. These analysts dismiss the nuclear freeze because they believe an accelerated nuclear build-up is necessary and that fighting a successful nuclear war is possible. With unintended irony, they even celebrate the recovery of Hiroshima and Nagasaki as proof that perhaps a nuclear conflict would not be all that bad. Their analysis also represents a case of unreflective analogy, for Hiroshima provides a stunning but nonetheless limited glimpse of the fearful consequences of the nuclear fire next time.

The paradox of Hiroshima is how horrifying it was there, and yet how small the bomb was then compared to the destructive power of a single modern missile, let alone the prospect of an all-out nuclear exchange. The terrible agony of Hiroshima was tempered by the fact that only one city was attacked at one time. Even in war torn Japan, there were other communities that eventually could send food, clothing, doctors, and at least some medical supplies. Of the survivors of the initial blast, tens of thousands more would have died slow deaths, as many of the wounded did, if there had been no place to flee and no help to be found. But in a general nuclear war four decades later, there will be little if any refuge or relief. San Diego would be incinerated with Los Angeles, Chicago with St. Louis, Boston with Providence. Even their suburbs would be burned to the ground; at best, the countryside would be contaminated, overrun by destruction, cut off from all communication and all supply lines. In the aftermath of a great natural disaster such as the Chicago fire or the earthquake in San Francisco, the rest of the nation could mount a massive rescue effort. But in a nuclear war, the greatest of all man-made disasters, it would be as though a nationwide fire or earthquake had struck. There would be nowhere to turn, no one for the tiny bands of devastated survivors to depend on. As one victim of Hiroshima has said, in such a war, "those who are alive will be dead."

So Hiroshima as history can teach the carnage of nuclear war, but it provides no prophecy of a postwar world. The United States and the Soviet Union have hundreds of cities with populations over 100,000 and a total of 17,000 strategic nuclear warheads—and in addition, 30,000 "smaller" warheads—available for the act of mutual obliteration. Today a Soviet-American nuclear conflict could mean thousands of Hiroshimas all at once, and this does not count the devastation in Europe, China, and elsewhere.

But the lesson of Hiroshima can reveal, to some extent, what the vastly bigger bombs of the 1980s would mean for the people of other potential Hiroshimas. And the example is important as an antidote to what psychiatrists call "psychic numbing" or "denial," the tendency to become habituated to the nuclear threat, to pretend that it does not exist, or that such a war could never really come.

We also have to discuss weapons policy and national defense in realistic terms. But we dare not lose sight of the human reality of weapons that could kill more people, sack more cities, burn more buildings, and inflict more suffering than in all the conflicts from the beginning of history until now. It may be useful to compare the size of American and Soviet missiles by setting up an array of models on a table in a congressional hearing room, but it is essential to remember that if the missiles those models represent are ever fired, there will be no table, no hearing room, and no Congress left to debate the aftermath.

In recent testimony on the Kennedy-Hatfield nuclear freeze resolution, one survivor of Hiroshima challenged the two most powerful nations on earth to have "a heart to do this, [to] freeze nuclear weapons." He understands that it would be a first step back from the madness which once nearly consumed his own life. He knows what a single B-29, carrying what would now be regarded as a baby bomb, did to his neighbors and his city. Different counts of the number killed at Hiroshima range as high as 300,000 out of a total population of 344,000. The city government offers an estimate of 200,000 killed. But it is certain that in the single minute after the *Enola Gay* (the B-29 which the pilot named for his mother,) dropped the "Thin Man" (the nickname of the first atomic bomb), at least 60,000 human beings were either dead or dying. The bomb dropped from the plane at 9:15 a.m.; by 9:16, a blast lasting less than a second raised the ground temperature 3000° centigrade, pushed the air pressure up to eight tons a square yard, and mounted a wind of fire that swept across the city. The fireball was half a mile wide; the mushroom cloud soared above 50,000 feet; from 270 miles away, the crew of the *Enola Gay* watched the cloud as it flashed an array of colors. What they saw was the first atomic rainbow.

But the event can only be truly told by those who were on the ground. The aggregate statistics of Hiroshima can cloud our consciousness as surely as the flashing mushroom cloud shielded the men on the *Enola Gay* from the human reality of the bomb they had just dropped. The Hiroshima victims, however, experienced a terrifying unreality. One of them has testified before Congress that weeks later, after he and others had first won the desperate struggle for bare survival, they began trying to comprehend that unreality; more than a third of a century has passed but the incomprehension has not. "I only can recount incidents," a survivor says.

Yet the "incidents" convey more powerfully than anything else what a nuclear war will mean to each of us. As Senator Paul Tsongas observed after hearing Hiroshima victims testify on the nuclear freeze, "I have never been so moved by a presentation. I think that we should take each member of the Senate and the House and those in the executive branch who have the power to stop this arms race and strap them to a chair and make them listen." If we did so, there might be less optimistic talk from war game theorists about how well Japan recovered from nuclear war.

Dr. Mitsuo Tomosawa, who was a fifteen-year-old student at Hiroshima in 1945, has said: "People who have never gone through the experience just cannot comprehend the misery, the suffering, the destruction." It is to be hoped that we will not have to learn these things the way the Hiroshima survivors did. But we can, and must, learn from their words. For the next nuclear war would be the second time for them. It would be the first, and probably the last time, for most of the rest of us. Though we cannot completely feel the pain of the Hiroshima victims, in a sense, the survivors have seen the future holocaust; they know its dark workings in human terms, and they have shared their painful memories with us.

Dr. Tomosawa and his fellow students were assigned to a work detail at an army supply depot three miles from the center of Hiroshima. On the morning of August 6, they were assembled in the depot courtyard when they heard the sound of B-29s. They assumed the planes were on a bombing run to Tokyo. A moment later, Tomosawa was surrounded "by a great flash of light, as if millions of flashbulbs were ignited at the same time." He ran blindly in the direction of an air-raid shelter. Then came the blast, and he was knocked unconscious.

When he came to, he could see again. And what he saw over the center of the city, what dominated his sight to the exclusion of all that was immediately around him, was the looming mushroom cloud, something unlike anything he had ever seen before. Then he rushed in abject fear back toward the air-raid shelter. After a few minutes, he walked out into the courtyard and found most of his friends buried under the debris of exploded walls and windows. Many of them were dead already; many other died while Tomosawa and friends who could still walk tried frantically to dig them out. Tomosawa wandered home through streets of corpses. One of the few people he saw alive was a dazed mother pushing a baby carriage; there was a hole in the baby's cheek, a piece of wood protruding from it.

Once he found his mother safe, Tomosawa went to a hospital to look for his closest friend. He was lying there with no one to care for him: "I couldn't recognize him because of his burns. He recognized me. He tried to smile at me, but that smile made him more grotesque. And soon, that evening, he died, without seeing his parents." Outside the hospital, the walking wounded filled the streets. Most of them had all their clothes burned off. Tomosawa couldn't tell whether they were men or women. "Practically all of them were walking with . . . their arms extended out, their hands hanging down, and their knees slightly bent, almost on tiptoes. There were large blisters on their bodies, with some fluid moving in the blisters. Staring ahead." They were in fact living, barely living zombies.

Others who had died were frozen by the blast in the last second of their lives, like the victims of the volcanic eruption of ancient Pompeii. Tomosawa saw people sitting and standing rigid in a streetcar, some with their hands still clinging to the overhead straps. He wondered why and then realized that their blackened forms had been seared into place. Other human forms stood at bus stops, or sat upright on their bicycles, frozen and dead, turned to statues of charcoal.

With fires raging through the city, even the open spaces were treacherous. Survivors like Tomosawa recall the windstorm created by the fire uprooting giant pine trees, hurling them five hundred feet into the air, and then the flaming trees smashing down into crowds of people. As the fires flickered out and night fell, the cries of the injured became a piercing wail. The city of Hiroshima, says Tomosawa, was "a desert of death."

Mrs. Hiroko Harris, who now lives in Baltimore and who was also a teenage student in Hiroshima, describes her experience: "People say after you die, you will have heaven or hell. But I don't believe that. I think hell was that day." What she recalls most of all was the intense heat. She was walking with her classmates toward a road repair project the students were working on when the explosion came. She felt that intense heat and feared that she would be burned to death. She jumped into the river, but even the water was hot. She swam across and climbed a hill, hoping to find her school still standing on the other side. At the top of the hill, she paused and looked back. Even the sky, she thought, was on fire.

A classmate, Shigeko Sasamori, fled in the opposite direction. In shock and unaware that she was injured, she stumbled on until she reached a burned-out house where she lay unconscious for four days. Finally, she heard her mother, wandering among the rubble, calling her name. She answered and her parents carried her home. They could not tell her face from the back of her head. Her father pulled off the blackened skin: "It was like a cream puff, yellow stuff underneath." She looked in a mirror: "I couldn't believe that was me. I had no eyebrows, no eyelashes—just bare face, with new soft skin tissues. The first time I realized that was me, I poured ice water over my body."

It took a month for her wounds to heal; in the years since 1945, she has had thirty-six operations to reconstruct her face. She concludes her story with words that should move the world: "I feel very strong about why I survived because many people died. And I feel I have a mission to survive, to tell the people, so it will never happen again. And if I can share my experience, to tell the people how horrible it is . . . But if I can scream, and other people scream, I hope everybody will hear this and understand it because I trust, I believe everybody has good hearts and everybody wants to care for each other, and we are God's children. And so we should be like God's children and love and care for each other."

Kimuko Laskey was sixteen years old and on duty sterilizing equipment in a Hiroshima hospital when the bomb was dropped. Now in Vancouver, British Columbia, she has brought her scars and her memories with her, and she, too, shared them with Americans during the congressional forum on the nuclear freeze. When the flash of the explosion came, she said, she tried to duck under a sturdy workbench built into the laboratory floor, but before she could move, she was blown out of the room. She felt she was "floating on the air, floating over this way and that way." She found herself on the hallway floor, then stood up slowly and went to the front of the hospital. The dead and the injured were everywhere. Out in the street, people were burned "like overcooked turkey." A friend in the hospital told Laskey her face was badly cut, and Laskey replied that her friend's was, too. They could not find any bandages, so they made them for each other out of curtain strips.

Since the heat in the hospital was unbearable, Laskey went to a nearby swimming pool. In the backyard, she saw "all orange up in the sky. You can't see blue anymore; you don't know what time of day it is. And that pool had so many people in it, over top one another, at the bottom the people were drowning; the top people was hot, trying to get in." She says that her hair was sweating, her dress was curling up. She went back to the street where she sat on a broken water pipe. She looked around and it was not only the sky, but the ground that glowed orange: "No way you can escape anymore."

When Laskey saw another friend, leaning on her parents, hobbling down the street on shredded ankles, she passed out. When she awakened, the orange glow had faded. Once again, there was "a beautiful blue sky," but there was something else as well: "Just everywhere was dead people." Laskey crawled back into the hospital, where doctors operated on her without anesthetic and sewed up her wounded face with a heavy needle. She crawled home, where her sister nursed her and her mother repeatedly, and walked four miles and back to draw cold water from the nearest spring. As she recovered, the family searched for her father. They found him in an air-raid shelter, the skin burned off his skeleton.

All the survivors share such stories and such sorrows. One was told how to look for his grandparents: go back to their house, "and if you find any greasy spots on the tile, you would find their bodies." Another survivor remembers people trapped under the debris of their houses, "the fire coming up near them, but no one can help, because everyone hurt." And one of the most pained of the Hiroshima witnesses can never forget the mother and her two children who were burned over 80 percent of their bodies. One of the children was crying out: "Please kill me. Please kill me. I cannot stand the pain." And the survivor thought: "I really did want to go there and kill that child."

The grim truth was that it was impossible to treat, or save, very many of the injured. Of the 298 doctors in Hiroshima, 270 had died. All but 135 of 1,780 nurses were killed. Only 3 of 45 hospitals still functioned at all. Only the "lucky" few were operated on, and those without anesthetic. And many of the people who thought they were fortunate to be alive soon found themselves fated to a lingering death. In the days after the bombing, there was an epidemic of nausea, vomiting, and radiation sickness; tens of thousands died within the next three weeks.

Dr. Stuart Finch, the chief of medicine at Cooper Medical Center in New Jersey, has described the process: "The bone marrow, gastrointestinal tract, and hair follicles were particularly sensitive to acute radiation effects. Damage to these tissues resulted in nausea, vomiting, diarrhea, severe infections, generalized bleeding, and extensive hair loss." In addition, a number of children in the wombs of Hiroshima mothers were exposed to substantial amounts of radiation. Dr. Finch reports: "Many were born with small head size and an appreciable number with mental retardation. Many children who were exposed experienced reduced growth and development." And thousands more perished in the next twenty years. The rate of leukemia climbed as high as forty times the normal rate. The incidence of other cancers multiplied three to six times. Hiroshima happened many years ago, but there is no end to the counting of the casualities. For those who still suffer and who still die from it, Hiroshima continues to happen every day.

The literally blinding light of the Hiroshima bomb also left people with lesions in the lens of their eyes and with cataracts. Many have progressively lost their sight; the vision of others is permanently shadowed. In a sense, their sickness is a metaphor for the blindness of the world to the nuclear danger. But no one who was in the city then can ever be blind to the danger now.

One of us, long before serving in the Senate, visited Hiroshima as a young naval officer only a month after the bombing. This is what Lieutenant (j.g.) Mark Hatfield saw: We were trying to get a comprehension of the heat that had been generated by the bomb, and we were walking on one of the bridges that was still standing. We noticed the shadows across the bridge from the balustrades, and yet we knew the sun was at high noon. Then we began to realize that the heat had actually made the shadows on solid concrete. As the heat swept across the bridge, those balustrades intercepted part of it, and made the stripes as though they had been painted on the concrete. We thought to ourselves: if that's what happened to the concrete of a bridge, what would this do to human flesh?

The history of Hiroshima is an agonizing story. But it is crucial to try to comprehend that agony so that it will never happen anywhere again. The campaign for a nuclear freeze depends in part on the rising public awareness about the hideous reality of nuclear war. Those of us in public life must persuade the nation, and citizens in local communities must persuade their neighbors, that nuclear war is not fightable, containable, winnable, or survivable. The only sensible purpose of defense policy is to prevent such a war, not to plan for fighting one. To remember Hiroshima is to resolve that the nuclear arms race must be stopped where it is now. Hiroshima should remind us of the imminent danger and stupidity of waiting for nuclear restraint while more and more megatons of explosive bombing power are buried in silos in the ground. It betrays the lesson of that first nuclear war to offer a freeze sometime in the future, or a freeze with preconditions, which would mean that both the United States and the Soviet Union could build more and more weapons, and negotiate at greater and greater length before entering into any agreement at all. Such a false freeze would not only increase nuclear weaponry but would add to the risk of a worldwide Hiroshima.

One survivor of Hiroshima, opening a shelter door minutes after the blast, exclaimed: "Oh, God." Almost the same words came from the co-pilot of the *Enola Gay*, who screamed "My God," as the bomb exploded from a tiny purple dot into a mammoth churning fireball. For both the pilot and the survivor, the words were a plea, a prayer, a cry of despair and hope. Thirty-seven years later, they summon us to freeze the nuclear arsenals of the great powers, to heed the Hiroshima survivors, and for their sake and for our own, at long last, to run the arms race in reverse.

2

THE NEXT NUCLEAR WAR
THE DEATH OF AN AMERICAN CITY

"If everyone had a profound and immediate sense of the actual consequences of nuclear war, we would be much more willing to confront and challenge leaders of all nations when they present narrow and self-serving arguments for the continuation of mutual nuclear terror."

—Carl Sagan

In the early days of World War II the scientists and military experts in the Manhattan Project were unsure what the explosive power of an atomic bomb would be as they raced to build it before Hitler's scientists developed one for Nazi Germany. The first atomic device, the experimental "Trinity" bomb tested at Alamogordo, New Mexico, in July 1945, turned out to be a 20-kiloton device—that is, it had the explosive equivalent of 20,000 tons of TNT. The bomb dropped on Hiroshima the next month was a 15-kiloton weapon.

Common sense might have suggested that one Hiroshima-size bomb was more than enough to take care of any target in even the most malevolent nuclear war strategy. But common sense was not, and never has been, the path of the nuclear arms race. The Soviet Union exploded its first nuclear device in 1949, and since then, both sides have pursued a practice that "more is better," and a policy that "if it can be built, it should be built." The advent of the hydrogen bomb in 1952 magnified the explosive capability of nuclear weapons; the second hydrogen bomb tested two years later at Bikini Atoll was a 15-megaton device, equivalent to 15 million tons of TNT, a thousand times the size of the Hiroshima bomb. Today atomic bombs are used to trigger hydrogen bombs. A common U.S. or Soviet intercontinental ballistic missile carries a 1-megaton warhead containing the explosive power of 1 million tons of TNT, or 67 Hiroshima bombs. Some U.S. warheads go as high as 9 megatons, equal to 600 Hiroshimas, and the Soviets have even tested a 50-megaton warhead, equal to 3300 Hiroshimas.

In the late 1960s both sides developed a technique to pack several nuclear warheads on a single missile, with each warhead capable of independent guidance to a separate target. These missiles deployed in the 1970s, are called "MIRV's" because the warheads are carried on "multiple independently targetable reentry vehicles." Our land-based Minuteman III missile has three such warheads, each containing up to a third of a megaton of TNT in explosive power. One of these missiles, therefore, could rain the equivalent of about 22 Hiroshima bombs on each of three different Soviet cities. The MX land-based missile now being developed by the Pentagon could carry up to 12 such warheads. In addition, the United States has 31 Poseidon submarines and 1 Trident submarine. However, under current Pentagon plans, 8 more Tridents will be built by the end of this decade. Most of the Poseidon submarines carry relatively smaller warheads of 40 kilotons, although some have now been fitted with larger Trident I missiles carrying 100-Kiloton warheads. A single Poseidon submarine, firing all 16 of its missiles, with 10 warheads each could smash 160 Soviet targets with the equivalent of nearly three Hiroshimas each.

The Soviets have a comparable attack capability. For example, some of their SS-18 missiles carry ten 1-megaton warheads; just one of these missiles could rain down on ten American targets the explosive power of 67 Hiroshimas each, and the Soviets have deployed over 300 SS-18s.

Total firepower on both sides of the arms race is staggering proof of the reality of overkill. This is the current state of the American and Soviet strategic nuclear arsenals capable of reaching each other's territory.

	U.S.	Soviet Union
Land-Based Intercontinental Ballistic Missiles (ICBMs)	1,052	1,398
Submarine-Launched Ballistic Missiles (SLBMs)	520	950
Long-Range Bombers	348	150
Total Delivery Vehicles (Launchers)	1,920	2,498
Total Warheads	9,400	7,500
Total Megatons	4,100	7,100

In addition, the two sides together have a total of approximately 30,000 nuclear warheads deployed for intermediate range use in regional conflicts and short range or "tactical" use against invading armies on the battlefield. Thus the total nuclear arsenals of the United States and the Soviet Union, including weapons of all ranges contain about 47,000 warheads.

By itself, the American arsenal of strategic weapons holds more destructive power than has been used in all the wars of ancient and modern history. U.S. forces are both vast and diversified:

Type of Launcher	Number of Launchers Deployed	Number of Warheads on Each Launcher	Yield Per Warhead (TNT Equivalent)	(Hiroshima Equivalent)
Intercontinental Ballistic Missiles (ICBMs)				
Titan II	52	1	9 megatons	600
Minuteman II	450	1	1 megaton	67
Minuteman III	550	3	170-350 kilotons	11-23
Submarine-Launched Ballistic Missiles (SLBMs)				
Poseidon	304	6-14	40 kilotons	3
Trident I	216	8	100 kilotons	7
Long-Range Bombers				
B-52 (1955)	90	4	1 megaton	67
B-52 (1962)	260	12-20	200 kilotons- 1 megaton	13-67

The Soviet strategic arsenal is comparable in destructive power:

Type of Launcher	Number of Launchers Deployed	Number of Warheads on Each Launcher	Yield Per Warhead (TNT Equivalent)	(Hiroshima Equivalent)
Intercontinental Ballistic Missiles (ICBMs)				
SS-11	520	1	1-2 megatons	67-133
SS-13	60	1	600 kilotons-1 megaton	40-67
SS-17	150	4	700 kilotons	47
SS-18	308	1-10	500 kilotons-2 megatons	33-133
SS-19	360	6	700 kilotons	47
Submarine-Launched Ballistic Missiles (SLBMs)				
SS-N-6	416	1	1 megaton	67
SS-N-8	280	1	2 megatons	133
SS-N-18	176	3 or 7	200-500 kilotons	13-33
Long-Range Bombers				
Bison	35	4	1 megaton	67
Bear	105	4	1 megaton	67

The overkill is obvious. Any imbalance between the two sides in one category of missiles, warheads, or megatons immediately pales beside the fact that each side has enough strategic nuclear weapons in its stockpile to inflict hundreds of thousands of Hiroshimas on the other. In their nuclear buildups over the past two decades, American and Soviet military planners have pursued different strategies to develop their present arsenals. One reason for the current imbalance in megatonnage, for example, is that the Soviets, less sophisticated technically, have found it necessary to build heavier missiles rather than lighter and more accurate ones. The American defense establishment choses not to construct heavier missiles, on the ground that with sufficient accuracy, a "smaller" bomb (for example, the equivalent of 25 Hiroshimas) would be equally effective in destroying any conceivable target. The "MAD" doctrine of nuclear deterrence (for "Mutual Assured Destruction") is a reality in 1982, just as it has been throughout the past two decades; the arsenals of the two sides are powerful enough to deter one another from launching any nuclear strike, because both sides realize they could face a retaliatory strike that would assure their own destruction. The essential point is that both sides already possess overkill piled upon overkill.

The United States and the Soviet Union have also pursued different strategies for the distribution of the weapons in their nuclear arsenals. Both rely on the "triad" of land-, sea-, and air-based weapons, but with different emphases on the legs of the triad. They rely much more heavily than we do on land-based missiles, and we rely more heavily than they do on submarines and bombers. According to the annual report of the Department of Defense for 1981, Soviet and U.S. nuclear warheads are distributed in these proportions:

Leg of Triad	United States	Soviet Union
Land-based (ICBMs)	24%	75%
Submarine-based (SLBMs)	50%	20%
Air-based (Long-Range Bombers)	26%	5%
	100%	100%

A number of authoritative studies have been conducted concerning the impact of the existing overkill, using various possible scenarios of nuclear attacks by the Soviet Union on the United States. In a large-scale assault, for example, the Soviets might fire 2000 warheads at American cities, not to mention the additional warheads aimed at our ICBM silos and other military and industrial targets. That means the Soviets could target 10 or 20 warheads (for good measure) on each city with a population over 1 million: New York, Chicago, Los Angeles, Philadelphia, Houston, and Detroit. They could allocate 5 or 10 warheads to each of the next hundred largest cities and still have enough left over to target a warhead on each of the next thousand cities. That would be enough to saturate every metropolitan area in the United States and reach towns with populations no larger than a few thousand. Every place of significant size would be totally destroyed, and even places like Mason City, Iowa, Florence, South Carolina and Ithaca, New York, could have Soviet nuclear warheads with their names on them. Most likely, in an all-out attack the 200 largest American cities would be obliterated in the first half hour. So would rural communities whose neighbors happen to be U.S. missile silos, bomber bases, or submarine ports.

What if a nuclear warhead hits your city or town? In 1979, the U.S. Arms Control and Disarmament Agency answered this question for each of the 545 urban areas in the United States with a population of 25,000 or more. In the aggregate, 132 million people live in these areas; the study found that the following percentages of people would be killed in a Soviet attack on these areas with various numbers of one-megaton warheads:

Number of Soviet Warheads Used To Attack U.S. Urban Areas	Percent of Total U. S. Urban Population Killed
100	27
200	40
300	50
400	58
500	64
1,000	84
1,500	94
2,000	98
2,500	100

The two accompanying tables list the deaths and injuries that will be suffered in each city under various levels of nuclear attack; in each case, it is assumed that the Soviet warhead would explode at a place and height that would produce the largest number of casualties in the area. The figures are based on census date describing where people reside in each area. If people are at work instead of at home when the bomb explodes, the casualty figures would be much higher since more people would be downtown and therefore closer to ground zero. The first table covers the 200 largest urban areas and assumes that they are hit by *two* warheads, each containing either a "baby" 50-kiloton bomb (equal to three Hiroshimas), a "regular size" 1-megaton bomb (equivalent to 67 Hiroshimas), or a "Big Bertha" 20-megaton bomb (equivalent to 1300 Hiroshimas). The second table covers the next

345 cities and assumes each is hit by a single warhead. In some cases the Soviets would not bother to use their biggest warhead since a smaller one would kill every human being in the area. In the past, the Soviets have deployed warheads up to 25 megatons, but their largest warheads currently deployed are 2-megaton weapons. When you hear talk about surviving a nuclear war, look up the city or town where you live and see whether you think you would be one of the survivors.

In 1979 the congressional Office of Technology Assessment (OTA), the congressional Joint Committee on Defense Production (now part of the Senate Banking Committee), and the U.S. Arms Control and Disarmament Agency published separate and detailed analyses of the effect of a nuclear attack on the United States. As shown in the table on page 44, which has been adapted from these studies, a nuclear explosion acts in three ways to kill and maim: by heat, blast, and radiation. The first injuries, delivered essentially at the speed of light, are caused by the intense light and heat radiated by the explosion and the fireball. The OTA study compared these consequences to the effect of a two-second flash of an enormous sunlamp. The fireball from a one-megaton blast would be a mile in diameter; to an observer 50 miles away, it would seem brighter than the noonday sun.

Approximately a third of the energy from a one-megaton explosion is released as heat and light. Those within five miles of ground zero will suffer horrible and often fatal third-degree skin burns. Anyone looking directly at the fireball from as far as 15 miles away on a clear day, and 60 miles on a clear night, will be blinded at least for several minutes; many will recover their sight, but many others will suffer permanent eye damage. As Dr. Jack Geiger, Professor of Community Medicine at City College of New York, told the Senate Health Subcommittee in 1980: "A person 40 miles away making a reflex glance at the fireball would, if he looked directly at it, suffer retinal burns and be blinded. People in Milwaukee would be blinded by the Chicago fireball. People in Baltimore would be blinded by the Washington fireball. People in San Jose would be blinded by the San Francisco fireball."

The intense heat generated by the blast will in turn ignite combustible materials in its path. Clothing will burst into flame; beds and furniture will be engulfed; serious fires will flare up in ruptured electrical and gas lines and damaged

Table 1. Number of persons killed and injured in large urban areas of the United States, each hit by two Soviet nuclear warheads. Warheads vary in size. (Dash indicates no survivors.)

Urban Area	Population	Fifty Kiloton Bomb (Three Hiroshimas)		One Megaton Bomb (67 Hiroshimas)		Twenty Megaton Bomb (1300 Hiroshimas)	
		Killed	Injured	Killed	Injured	Killed	Injured
Abilene, Kansas	94,000	60,000	25,000	91,000	3,000	94,000	—
Akron, Ohio	463,000	87,000	125,000	325,000	97,000	460,000	3,000
Albany, Georgia	83,000	42,000	25,000	81,000	2,000	83,000	—
Albany, New York	457,000	101,000	107,000	306,000	102,000	446,000	11,000
Albuquerque, New Mexico	367,000	82,000	120,000	314,000	42,000	364,000	3,000
Allentown, Pennsylvania	276,000	90,000	88,000	223,000	46,000	276,000	—
Alton, Illinois	98,000	41,000	31,000	87,000	9,000	98,000	—
Altoona, Pennsylvania	87,000	46,000	18,000	85,000	2,000	87,000	—
Amarillo, Texas	129,000	54,000	35,000	122,000	6,000	129,000	—
Anchorage, Alaska	132,000	53,000	40,000	126,000	6,000	132,000	—
Ann Arbor, Michigan	188,000	78,000	65,000	179,000	8,000	188,000	—
Appleton, Wisconsin	136,000	65,000	28,000	115,000	15,000	135,000	1,000
Atlanta, Georgia	1,298,000	76,000	88,000	548,000	386,000	1,169,000	108,000
Augusta, Georgia	162,000	47,000	50,000	140,000	20,000	162,000	—
Aurora, Illinois	153,000	68,000	46,000	146,000	7,000	151,000	2,000
Austin, Texas	334,000	69,000	108,000	292,000	35,000	333,000	1,000
Bakersfield, California	186,000	73,000	61,000	175,000	11,000	186,000	—
Baltimore, Maryland	1,484,000	98,000	294,000	928,000	391,000	1,458,000	25,000

17

Urban Area	Population	Fifty Kiloton Bomb (Three Hiroshimas)		One Megaton Bomb (67 Hiroshimas)		Twenty Megaton Bomb (1300 Hiroshimas)	
		Killed	Injured	Killed	Injured	Killed	Injured
Baton Rouge, Louisiana	278,000	81,000	75,000	230,000	41,000	278,000	—
Beaumont, Texas	110,000	44,000	42,000	104,000	6,000	110,000	—
Billings, Montana	82,000	55,000	19,000	81,000	1,000	82,000	—
Biloxi, Mississippi	122,000	39,000	32,000	110,000	11,000	122,000	—
Binghamton, New York	163,000	58,000	53,000	148,000	12,000	163,000	—
Birmingham, Alabama	549,000	74,000	114,000	318,000	143,000	534,000	14,000
Boise City, Idaho	115,000	54,000	46,000	115,000	—	115,000	—
Boston, Massachusetts	2,884,000	210,000	393,000	1,033,000	789,000	2,315,000	398,000
Boulder, Colorado	99,000	64,000	26,000	99,000	—	99,000	—
Buffalo, New York	939,000	201,000	249,000	664,000	215,000	934,000	4,000
Canton, Ohio	237,000	77,000	60,000	210,000	21,000	234,000	3,000
Cedar Rapids, Iowa	129,000	56,000	39,000	118,000	11,000	129,000	—
Champaign, Illinois	104,000	66,000	27,000	103,000	1,000	104,000	—
Charleston, South Carolina	219,000	62,000	53,000	177,000	33,000	214,000	5,000
Charleston, West Virginia	145,000	47,000	35,000	117,000	15,000	144,000	1,000
Charlotte, North Carolina	313,000	77,000	92,000	255,000	51,000	313,000	—
Chattanooga, Tennessee	216,000	40,000	71,000	180,000	32,000	215,000	1,000

Chicago, Illinois	6,659,000	241,000	789,000	2,096,000	1,535,000	4,874,000	1,186,000
Cincinnati, Ohio	1,145,000	75,000	234,000	571,000	356,000	1,088,000	47,000
Cleveland, Ohio	1,890,000	139,000	165,000	937,000	422,000	1,613,000	193,000
Colorado Spring, Colorado	254,000	49,000	75,000	223,000	25,000	253,000	1,000
Columbia, South Carolina	245,000	65,000	69,000	205,000	32,000	244,000	1,000
Columbus, Georgia	186,000	37,000	58,000	160,000	19,000	185,000	1,000
Columbus, Ohio	801,000	89,000	179,000	515,000	217,000	795,000	6,000
Concord, California	302,000	64,000	77,000	231,000	57,000	295,000	7,000
Corpus Christi, Texas	189,000	77,000	61,000	180,000	9,000	189,000	—
Dallas, Texas	2,087,000	89,000	168,000	572,000	507,000	1,788,000	246,000
Davenport, Iowa	250,000	86,000	78,000	224,000	21,000	250,000	—
Dayton, Ohio	702,000	86,000	110,000	381,000	162,000	670,000	26,000
Daytona Beach, Florida	126,000	51,000	36,000	119,000	5,000	126,000	—
Decatur, Illinois	96,000	50,000	32,000	95,000	1,000	96,000	—
Denver, Colorado	1,162,000	78,000	167,000	618,000	358,000	1,137,000	24,000
Des Moines, Iowa	269,000	76,000	77,000	228,000	38,000	269,000	—
Detroit, Michigan	3,858,000	105,000	272,000	1,243,000	1,077,000	3,212,000	536,000
Duluth, Minnesota	116,000	44,000	32,000	99,000	14,000	116,000	—
Durham, North Carolina	103,000	57,000	31,000	101,000	2,000	103,000	—
Easton, Pennsylvania	87,000	50,000	25,000	84,000	3,000	87,000	—
El Paso, Texas	385,000	80,000	85,000	288,000	69,000	383,000	2,000
Erie, Pennsylvania	174,000	91,000	48,000	163,000	11,000	174,000	—
Eugene, Oregon	154,000	56,000	45,000	141,000	12,000	154,000	—

Urban Area	Population	Fifty Kiloton Bomb (Three Hiroshimas) Killed	Injured	One Megaton Bomb (67 Hiroshimas) Killed	Injured	Twenty Megaton Bomb (1300 Hiroshimas) Killed	Injured
Evansville, Indiana	138,000	68,000	56,000	132,000	6,000	138,000	—
Fargo, North Dakota	92,000	58,000	27,000	91,000	1,000	92,000	—
Fayetteville, North Carolina	174,000	53,000	54,000	157,000	15,000	173,000	1,000
Flint, Michigan	295,000	75,000	98,000	257,000	32,000	294,000	1,000
Fort Smith, Arkansas	83,000	38,000	23,000	76,000	6,000	83,000	—
Fort Wayne, Indiana	228,000	75,000	76,000	205,000	20,000	228,000	—
Fresno, California	289,000	63,000	103,000	267,000	19,000	289,000	—
Gainesville, Florida	88,000	54,000	23,000	85,000	3,000	88,000	—
Gastonia, North Carolina	102,000	43,000	27,000	94,000	7,000	101,000	1,000
Grand Rapids, Michigan	359,000	87,000	102,000	285,000	60,000	356,000	3,000
Green Bay, Wisconsin	144,000	88,000	32,000	142,000	1,000	144,000	—
Greensboro, North Carolina	155,000	49,000	58,000	147,000	8,000	155,000	—
Greenville, South Carolina	185,000	38,000	74,000	161,000	21,000	184,000	1,000
Harrisburg, Pennsylvania	253,000	69,000	61,000	198,000	38,000	252,000	1,000
Hartford, Connecticut	651,000	144,000	118,000	390,000	144,000	612,000	29,000
Honolulu, Hawaii	483,000	141,000	98,000	384,000	75,000	476,000	6,000

City	1,807,000	78,000	201,000	782,000	584,000	1,706,000	89,000
Houston, Texas	1,807,000	78,000	201,000	782,000	584,000	1,706,000	89,000
Huntington, West Virginia	161,000	61,000	31,000	133,000	22,000	159,000	2,000
Huntsville, Alabama	143,000	48,000	46,000	130,000	12,000	143,000	—
Indianapolis, Indiana	780,000	61,000	82,000	484,000	206,000	753,000	25,000
Jackson, Mississippi	191,000	71,000	54,000	169,000	20,000	191,000	—
Jacksonville, Florida	547,000	83,000	111,000	363,000	144,000	542,000	5,000
Johnstown, Pennsylvania	90,000	42,000	26,000	89,000	1,000	90,000	—
Joliet, Illinois	166,000	80,000	56,000	161,000	5,000	166,000	—
Kailua, Hawaii	94,000	52,000	27,000	92,000	2,000	94,000	—
Kalamazoo, Michigan	134,000	63,000	40,000	127,000	5,000	134,000	—
Kansas City, Missouri	1,027,000	94,000	121,000	495,000	326,000	991,000	33,000
Kenosha, Wisconsin	83,000	71,000	10,000	83,000	—	83,000	—
Killeen, Texas	93,000	69,000	19,000	93,000	—	93,000	1,000
Knoxville, Tennessee	209,000	62,000	73,000	175,000	29,000	208,000	—
Lafayette, Louisiana	102,000	52,000	34,000	98,000	4,000	102,000	—
Lake Charles, Louisiana	96,000	46,000	32,000	94,000	1,000	96,000	—
Lakeland, Florida	84,000	48,000	20,000	81,000	3,000	84,000	—
Lancaster, Pennsylvania	110,000	70,000	27,000	108,000	2,000	110,000	—
Lansing, Michigan	245,000	85,000	75,000	215,000	23,000	245,000	—
Las Vegas, Nevada	292,000	62,000	94,000	243,000	41,000	292,000	—
Lawrence, Maine	117,000	67,000	36,000	113,000	4,000	117,000	—
Lawton, Oklahoma	93,000	50,000	24,000	92,000	1,000	93,000	—
Lexington, Kentucky	178,000	81,000	65,000	172,000	6,000	178,000	—
Lincoln, Nebraska	168,000	67,000	71,000	165,000	3,000	168,000	—

Urban Area	Population	Fifty Kiloton Bomb (Three Hiroshimas)		One Megaton Bomb (67 Hiroshimas)		Twenty Megaton Bomb (1300 Hiroshimas)	
		Killed	Injured	Killed	Injured	Killed	Injured
Little Rock, Arkansas	246,000	55,000	60,000	196,000	40,000	245,000	1,000
Los Angeles, California	8,664,000	130,000	370,000	1,489,000	1,808,000	5,736,000	2,041,000
Louisville, Kentucky	717,000	123,000	128,000	442,000	197,000	709,000	8,000
Lubbock, Texas	163,000	52,000	65,000	157,000	5,000	163,000	—
Macon, Georgia	125,000	53,000	41,000	119,000	5,000	125,000	—
Madison, Wisconsin	209,000	68,000	54,000	175,000	28,000	209,000	—
Manchester, New Hampshire	99,000	61,000	28,000	95,000	4,000	99,000	—
Memphis, Tennessee	698,000	79,000	196,000	477,000	162,000	693,000	5,000
Miami, Florida	2,320,000	125,000	179,000	801,000	718,000	2,005,000	231,000
Milwaukee, Wisconsin	1,137,000	149,000	226,000	693,000	293,000	1,113,000	21,000
Minneapolis, Minnesota	1,577,000	71,000	179,000	761,000	436,000	1,469,000	98,000
Mobile, Alabama	276,000	85,000	72,000	224,000	40,000	275,000	1,000
Modesto, California	128,000	73,000	40,000	126,000	1,000	128,000	—
Monroe, Louisiana	107,000	37,000	44,000	103,000	4,000	107,000	—
Montgomery, Alabama	158,000	57,000	58,000	155,000	3,000	158,000	—
Muncie, Indiana	87,000	57,000	24,000	84,000	3,000	87,000	—
Muskegon, Illinois	101,000	47,000	29,000	100,000	1,000	101,000	—
Nashville, Tennessee	398,000	66,000	98,000	271,000	97,000	394,000	4,000
New Bedford, Connecticut	135,000	77,000	43,000	135,000	1,000	136,000	—

New Orleans, Louisiana	1,015,000	132,000	175,000	684,000	241,000	1,006,000	8,000
New York, New York	16,323,000	693,000	1,053,000	3,070,000	4,095,000	9,583,000	3,654,000
Newburgh, New York	81,000	46,000	16,000	78,000	3,000	81,000	—
Newport News, Virginia	267,000	73,000	65,000	200,000	51,000	267,000	—
Niagara Falls, New York	110,000	68,000	25,000	105,000	4,000	110,000	—
Norfolk, Virginia	688,000	88,000	116,000	398,000	204,000	668,000	18,000
Odessa, Texas	87,000	58,000	24,000	86,000	1,000	87,000	—
Ogden, Utah	96,000	51,000	38,000	93,000	3,000	96,000	—
Oklahoma City, Oklahoma	499,000	61,000	101,000	309,000	149,000	496,000	3,000
Omaha, Nebraska	524,000	78,000	135,000	369,000	125,000	522,000	2,000
Orlando, Florida	407,000	57,000	93,000	278,000	95,000	404,000	3,000
Oxnard, California	202,000	72,000	37,000	182,000	17,000	201,000	1,000
Pensacola, Florida	182,000	62,000	48,000	159,000	19,000	182,000	—
Peoria, Illinois	208,000	80,000	54,000	181,000	21,000	208,000	—
Petersburg, Virginia	104,000	46,000	31,000	98,000	5,000	104,000	—
Philadelphia, Pennsylvania	4,557,000	226,000	298,000	1,456,000	1,258,000	3,498,000	674,000
Phoenix, Arizona	996,000	74,000	128,000	552,000	288,000	955,000	32,000
Pittsburgh, Pennsylvania	1,716,000	134,000	198,000	717,000	505,000	1,485,000	180,000
Portland, Maine	115,000	54,000	29,000	112,000	3,000	115,000	—
Portland, Oregon	782,000	81,000	199,000	516,000	191,000	776,000	5,000
Providence, Rhode Island	892,000	99,000	122,000	457,000	210,000	797,000	73,000
Provo, Utah	103,000	70,000	24,000	101,000	2,000	103,000	—

Urban Area	Population	Fifty Kiloton Bomb (Three Hiroshimas) Killed	Injured	One Megaton Bomb (67 Hiroshimas) Killed	Injured	Twenty Megaton Bomb (1300 Hiroshimas) Killed	Injured
Pueblo, Colorado	109,000	58,000	35,000	108,000	1,000	109,000	—
Racine, Wisconsin	121,000	80,000	31,000	120,000	1,000	121,000	—
Raleigh, North Carolina	183,000	60,000	55,000	160,000	20,000	183,000	—
Reading, Pennsylvania	178,000	80,000	52,000	165,000	12,000	178,000	—
Reno, Nevada	123,000	56,000	44,000	121,000	2,000	123,000	—
Richmond, Virginia	477,000	96,000	108,000	343,000	108,000	472,000	5,000
Riverside, California	541,000	57,000	60,000	302,000	156,000	514,000	23,000
Roanoke, Virginia	168,000	43,000	59,000	148,000	16,000	168,000	—
Rochester, New York	599,000	161,000	146,000	444,000	112,000	597,000	2,000
Rockford, Illinois	198,000	80,000	67,000	186,000	10,000	198,000	—
Sacramento, California	745,000	75,000	143,000	452,000	208,000	727,000	16,000
Saginaw, Michigan	147,000	83,000	44,000	145,000	2,000	147,000	—
St. Louis, Missouri	1,800,000	125,000	235,000	792,000	550,000	1,639,000	136,000
St. Petersburg, Florida	651,000	61,000	123,000	442,000	158,000	641,000	8,000
Salem, Oregon	113,000	55,000	30,000	109,000	4,000	113,000	—
Salt Lake City, Utah	483,000	100,000	119,000	345,000	114,000	483,000	—
San Antonio, Texas	865,000	64,000	130,000	581,000	204,000	862,000	3,000
San Diego, California	1,347,000	138,000	134,000	649,000	426,000	1,301,000	43,000
San Francisco, California	3,613,000	177,000	322,000	1,096,000	665,000	2,726,000	705,000
San Rafael, California	207,000	47,000	40,000	154,000	30,000	203,000	4,000
Santa Barbara, California	151,000	52,000	39,000	141,000	9,000	150,000	1,000

Santa Cruz, California	98,000	52,000	27,000	93,000	4,000	98,000	—
Santa Rosa, California	84,000	55,000	21,000	81,000	3,000	84,000	—
Sarasota, Florida	224,000	59,000	65,000	189,000	29,000	222,000	2,000
Savannah, Georgia	152,000	69,000	42,000	141,000	9,000	152,000	—
Scranton, Pennsylvania	374,000	90,000	94,000	283,000	64,000	343,000	30,000
Seaside, California	135,000	55,000	34,000	115,000	15,000	135,000	—
Seattle, Washington	1,213,000	90,000	141,000	530,000	338,000	1,051,000	113,000
Shreveport, Louisiana	226,000	44,000	97,000	202,000	22,000	226,000	—
Sioux City, Iowa	90,000	52,000	28,000	88,000	2,000	90,000	—
South Bend, Indiana	282,000	64,000	62,000	226,000	40,000	278,000	3,000
Spokane, Washington	254,000	70,000	72,000	214,000	34,000	254,000	—
Springfield, Illinois	131,000	68,000	41,000	126,000	5,000	131,000	—
Springfield, Maine	415,000	101,000	87,000	311,000	69,000	413,000	2,000
Springfield, Missouri	127,000	51,000	49,000	127,000	—	127,000	—
Springfield, Ohio	95,000	62,000	20,000	93,000	2,000	95,000	—
Stockton, California	164,000	65,000	60,000	156,000	8,000	164,000	—
Syracuse, New York	355,000	112,000	92,000	289,000	49,000	351,000	4,000
Tacoma, Washington	299,000	72,000	54,000	236,000	54,000	297,000	2,000
Tallahassee, Florida	95,000	61,000	25,000	93,000	2,000	95,000	—
Tampa, Florida	396,000	78,000	54,000	300,000	69,000	394,000	2,000
Toledo, Ohio	470,000	98,000	113,000	356,000	92,000	466,000	4,000
Topeka, Kansas	118,000	43,000	45,000	115,000	3,000	118,000	—
Tucson, Arizona	379,000	75,000	60,000	296,000	70,000	378,000	1,000
Tulsa, Oklahoma	369,000	55,000	79,000	289,000	62,000	368,000	1,000
Tuscaloosa, Alabama	88,000	49,000	26,000	85,000	3,000	88,000	—

Urban Area	Population	Fifty Kiloton Bomb (Three Hiroshimas) Killed	Injured	One Megaton Bomb (67 Hiroshimas) Killed	Injured	Twenty Megaton Bomb (1300 Hiroshimas) Killed	Injured
Utica, New York	130,000	64,000	39,000	128,000	2,000	130,000	—
Vallejo, California	85,000	55,000	25,000	85,000	—	85,000	—
Vancouver, Washington	85,000	46,000	30,000	84,000	1,000	85,000	—
Waco, Texas	113,000	47,000	43,000	109,000	4,000	113,000	—
Washington, DC	2,554,000	201,000	278,000	957,000	836,000	2,387,000	147,000
Waterbury, Connecticut	138,000	75,000	30,000	130,000	7,000	138,000	—
Waterloo, Iowa	107,000	53,000	33,000	98,000	8,000	107,000	—
West Palm Beach, Florida	358,000	72,000	44,000	234,000	71,000	340,000	13,000
Wheeling, West Virginia	114,000	33,000	35,000	95,000	17,000	112,000	2,000
Wichita, Kansas	290,000	58,000	97,000	252,000	30,000	289,000	1,000
Wichita Falls, Texas	98,000	32,000	37,000	87,000	10,000	98,000	—
Winston-Salem, North Carolina	152,000	54,000	49,000	142,000	10,000	152,000	—
Worcester, Massachusetts	231,000	86,000	68,000	206,000	21,000	231,000	—
York, Pennsylvania	112,000	65,000	30,000	109,000	3,000	112,000	—
Youngstown, Ohio	387,000	59,000	91,000	290,000	73,000	378,000	8,000

Table 2. Number of persons killed and injured in smaller urban areas of the United States, each hit by one Soviet nuclear warhead. Warheads vary in size.

Urban Area	Population	Fifty Kiloton Bomb (Three Hiroshimas)		One Megaton Bomb (67 Hiroshimas)		Twenty Megaton Bomb (1300 Hiroshimas)	
		Killed	Injured	Killed	Injured	Killed	Injured
Aberdeen, South Dakota	27,000	21,000	5,000	27,000	—	27,000	—
Aberdeen, Washington	30,000	14,000	8,000	29,000	1,000	30,000	—
Alexandria, Louisiana	71,000	22,000	26,000	67,000	4,000	71,000	—
Alliance, Ohio	30,000	25,000	4,000	30,000	—	30,000	—
Ames, Iowa	44,000	25,000	13,000	44,000	—	44,000	—
Amsterdam, New York	26,000	20,000	6,000	26,000	—	26,000	—
Anderson, Indiana	63,000	31,000	19,000	62,000	1,000	63,000	—
Anderson, South Carolina	47,000	23,000	14,000	45,000	2,000	47,000	—
Annapolis, Maryland	52,000	30,000	15,000	51,000	1,000	52,000	—
Anniston, Alabama	47,000	24,000	11,000	45,000	2,000	47,000	—
Ansonia, Connecticut	55,000	21,000	18,000	49,000	6,000	55,000	—
Antioch, Ohio	74,000	22,000	14,000	57,000	13,000	74,000	—
Asheville, North Carolina	74,000	19,000	24,000	64,000	10,000	74,000	—
Ashtabula, Ohio	32,000	15,000	12,000	32,000	—	32,000	—
Athens, Georgia	50,000	30,000	14,000	50,000	—	50,000	—
Atlantic City, New Jersey	74,000	39,000	12,000	68,000	5,000	74,000	—

Urban Area	Population	Fifty Kiloton Bomb (Three Hiroshimas)		One Megaton Bomb (67 Hiroshimas)		Twenty Megaton Bomb (1300 Hiroshimas)	
		Killed	Injured	Killed	Injured	Killed	Injured
Auburn, New York	37,000	26,000	9,000	37,000	—	37,000	—
Austin, Minnesota	25,000	19,000	4,000	25,000	—	25,000	—
Bangor, Maine	38,000	28,000	6,000	37,000	1,000	38,000	—
Bartlesville, Oklahoma	32,000	13,000	8,000	32,000	—	32,000	—
Battle Creek, Michigan	74,000	33,000	21,000	70,000	3,000	74,000	—
Bay City, Michigan	71,000	30,000	27,000	70,000	1,000	71,000	—
Baytown, Texas	41,000	26,000	10,000	41,000	—	41,000	—
Bellingham, Washington	46,000	24,000	13,000	46,000	—	46,000	—
Beloit, Wisconsin	48,000	28,000	11,000	48,000	—	48,000	—
Benton Harbor, Michigan	49,000	24,000	16,000	49,000	—	49,000	—
Biddeford, Maine	34,000	22,000	7,000	33,000	1,000	34,000	—
Big Spring, Texas	29,000	21,000	6,000	29,000	—	29,000	—
Bismarck, North Dakota	43,000	30,000	11,000	43,000	—	43,000	—
Bloomington, Illinois	78,000	49,000	19,000	77,000	1,000	78,000	—
Bloomington, Indiana	53,000	34,000	13,000	53,000	—	53,000	—
Blytheville, Arkansas	26,000	18,000	4,000	26,000	—	26,000	—
Bountiful, Vermont	52,000	31,000	13,000	52,000	—	52,000	—
Bowie, Maryland	39,000	24,000	10,000	39,000	—	39,000	—
Bowling Green, Kentucky	40,000	24,000	11,000	40,000	—	40,000	—
Bremerton, Washington	65,000	25,000	22,000	62,000	3,000	65,000	—
Bristol, Virginia	42,000	20,000	13,000	41,000	1,000	42,000	—

Brownsville, Texas	56,000	37,000	12,000	56,000	—	56,000
Brunswick, Georgia	32,000	15,000	10,000	31,000	1,000	32,000
Bryan, Texas	69,000	23,000	13,000	63,000	5,000	69,000
Burlington, Iowa	34,000	24,000	8,000	34,000	—	34,000
Burlington, North Carolina	67,000	29,000	17,000	58,000	7,000	67,000
Burlington, Vermont	60,000	29,000	17,000	57,000	2,000	60,000
Butler, Pennsylvania	35,000	24,000	7,000	35,000	—	35,000
Butte, Montana	41,000	25,000	10,000	41,000	—	41,000
Camarillo, California	32,000	20,000	8,000	32,000	—	32,000
Cape Girardeau, Missouri	29,000	21,000	6,000	29,000	—	29,000
Carbondale, Illinois	29,000	20,000	7,000	29,000	—	29,000
Carlisle, Pennsylvania	26,000	21,000	5,000	26,000	—	26,000
Carpentersville, Illinois	34,000	23,000	7,000	34,000	—	34,000
Casper, Wyoming	48,000	25,000	13,000	48,000	—	48,000
Chapel Hill, North Carolina	43,000	28,000	11,000	43,000	—	43,000
Charlottesville, Virginia	61,000	31,000	19,000	61,000	—	61,000
Cheyenne, Wyoming	52,000	24,000	17,000	51,000	1,000	52,000
Chico, California	43,000	31,000	9,000	43,000	—	43,000
Chillicothe, Ohio	27,000	18,000	7,000	27,000	—	27,000
Clarksburg, West Virginia	35,000	24,000	8,000	35,000	—	35,000
Clarksville, Tennessee	38,000	12,000	11,000	34,000	4,000	38,000
Cleveland, Tennessee	37,000	18,000	11,000	36,000	1,000	37,000
Clinton, Wisconsin	37,000	19,000	12,000	37,000	—	37,000
Clovis, New Mexico	35,000	23,000	8,000	35,000	—	35,000
Columbia, Missouri	51,000	34,000	13,000	51,000	—	51,000

Urban Area	Population	Fifty Kiloton Bomb (Three Hiroshimas) Killed	Injured	One Megaton Bomb (67 Hiroshimas) Killed	Injured	Twenty Megaton Bomb (1300 Hiroshimas) Killed	Injured
Columbus, Indiana	26,000	17,000	7,000	26,000	—	26,000	—
Columbus, Mississippi	30,000	22,000	5,000	30,000	—	30,000	—
Concord, New Hampshire	30,000	17,000	9,000	30,000	—	30,000	—
Coos Bay, Oregon	28,000	10,000	7,000	27,000	1,000	28,000	—
Corvallis, Oregon	43,000	34,000	7,000	43,000	—	43,000	—
Cumberland, Maryland	42,000	22,000	12,000	41,000	1,000	42,000	—
Dalton, Georgia	30,000	21,000	7,000	30,000	—	30,000	—
Danbury, Connecticut	45,000	29,000	11,000	45,000	—	45,000	—
Danville, Illinois	50,000	22,000	16,000	49,000	1,000	50,000	—
Danville, Virginia	49,000	21,000	17,000	49,000	—	49,000	—
Davis, California	33,000	24,000	7,000	33,000	—	33,000	—
Decatur, Alabama	41,000	19,000	14,000	41,000	—	41,000	—
DeKalb, Illinois	34,000	26,000	7,000	34,000	—	34,000	—
Denison, Texas	25,000	18,000	5,000	25,000	—	25,000	—
Denton, Texas	50,000	34,000	11,000	50,000	—	50,000	—
Dothan, Alabama	47,000	35,000	9,000	47,000	—	47,000	—
Dover, Delaware	34,000	19,000	8,000	33,000	1,000	34,000	—
Dubuque, Iowa	65,000	35,000	20,000	65,000	—	65,000	—
Dunkirk, New York	30,000	13,000	12,000	30,000	—	30,000	—
East Liverpool, Ohio	34,000	17,000	11,000	34,000	—	34,000	—
Eau Claire, Wisconsin	64,000	33,000	16,000	63,000	1,000	64,000	—

	25,000	16,000	7,000	25,000	—	25,000	
El Dorado, Arkansas	25,000	16,000	7,000	25,000	—	25,000	
Elgin, Illinois	71,000	42,000	18,000	70,000	1,000	71,000	
Elmira, New York	72,000	28,000	22,000	64,000	7,000	72,000	
Enid, Oklahoma	46,000	25,000	15,000	46,000	—	46,000	
Escondido, California	55,000	27,000	18,000	55,000	—	55,000	
Eureka, California	36,000	21,000	10,000	36,000	—	36,000	
Fairbanks, Alaska	35,000	18,000	10,000	34,000	1,000	35,000	
Fairfield, California	42,000	27,000	11,000	42,000	—	42,000	
Fairmont, West Virginia	28,000	19,000	7,000	28,000	—	28,000	
Fayetteville, Arkansas	36,000	29,000	6,000	36,000	—	36,000	
Findley, Ohio	38,000	23,000	11,000	38,000	—	38,000	
Fitchburg, Massachusetts	76,000	29,000	17,000	71,000	5,000	76,000	
Flagstaff, Arizona	40,000	22,000	8,000	39,000	1,000	40,000	
Florence, Alabama	73,000	18,000	14,000	60,000	10,000	73,000	
Florence, South Carolina	38,000	20,000	11,000	38,000	—	38,000	
Fond du Lac, Wisconsin	41,000	37,000	3,000	41,000	—	41,000	
Fort Collins, Colorado	67,000	39,000	19,000	67,000	—	67,000	
Fort Dodge, Iowa	30,000	20,000	7,000	30,000	—	30,000	
Fort Knox, Kentucky	37,000	26,000	7,000	37,000	—	37,000	
Fort Myers, Florida	64,000	25,000	15,000	56,000	6,000	64,000	
Fort Pierce, Florida	50,000	37,000	9,000	50,000	—	50,000	
Fort Walton Beach, Florida	51,000	22,000	17,000	50,000	1,000	51,000	
Frederick, Maryland	30,000	29,000	1,000	30,000	—	30,000	

Urban Area	Population	Fifty Kiloton Bomb (Three Hiroshimas) Killed	Injured	One Megaton Bomb (67 Hiroshimas) Killed	Injured	Twenty Megaton Bomb (1300 Hiroshimas) Killed	Injured
Freeport, Illinois	27,000	21,000	4,000	27,000	—	27,000	—
Gadsden, Alabama	55,000	13,000	12,000	51,000	3,000	55,000	—
Gainesville, Georgia	30,000	21,000	7,000	30,000	—	30,000	—
Galesburg, Illinois	37,000	30,000	6,000	37,000	—	37,000	—
Galveston, Texas	70,000	34,000	19,000	68,000	2,000	70,000	—
Glassboro, New Jersey	33,000	18,000	8,000	31,000	1,000	33,000	—
Glens Falls, New York	59,000	23,000	16,000	55,000	4,000	59,000	—
Gloucester, Massachusetts	26,000	20,000	5,000	26,000	—	26,000	—
Gloversville, New York	36,000	19,000	7,000	35,000	1,000	36,000	—
Goldsboro, North Carolina	42,000	22,000	10,000	40,000	2,000	42,000	—
Grand Forks, North Dakota	48,000	33,000	10,000	48,000	—	48,000	—
Grand Island, Nebraska	35,000	30,000	4,000	35,000	—	35,000	—
Grand Junction, Colorado	35,000	22,000	10,000	35,000	—	35,000	—
Great Falls, Montana	74,000	31,000	20,000	68,000	5,000	74,000	—
Greeley, Colorado	53,000	34,000	15,000	53,000	—	53,000	—
Greensburg, Pennsylvania	39,000	26,000	9,000	39,000	—	39,000	—
Greenville, Mississippi	44,000	32,000	9,000	44,000	—	44,000	—

Greenville, North Carolina	32,000	25,000	6,000	32,000	—	32,000
Greenwood, South Carolina	27,000	17,000	7,000	27,000	—	27,000
Griffin, Georgia	38,000	27,000	7,000	38,000	—	38,000
Hagerstown, Maryland	51,000	30,000	13,000	50,000	1,000	51,000
Hanover, Pennsylvania	26,000	18,000	6,000	26,000	—	26,000
Harlingen, Texas	38,000	28,000	8,000	38,000	—	38,000
Hattiesburg, Mississippi	48,000	23,000	15,000	47,000	1,000	48,000
Haverhill, Massachusetts	41,000	25,000	10,000	41,000	—	41,000
Hazleton, Pennsylvania	35,000	27,000	6,000	35,000	—	35,000
Hemet, California	32,000	20,000	7,000	31,000	1,000	32,000
Hickory, North Carolina	45,000	21,000	11,000	43,000	2,000	45,000
High Point, North Carolina	69,000	32,000	20,000	67,000	2,000	69,000
Hobbs, New Mexico	29,000	24,000	4,000	29,000	—	29,000
Holland, Indiana	47,000	27,000	9,000	42,000	4,000	47,000
Homestead, Florida	50,000	20,000	7,000	41,000	8,000	50,000
Hopkinsville, Kentucky	35,000	22,000	9,000	35,000	—	35,000
Hot Springs, Arkansas	41,000	23,000	13,000	41,000	—	41,000
Houma, Louisiana	47,000	25,000	13,000	46,000	1,000	47,000
Hutchinson, Kansas	41,000	28,000	8,000	41,000	—	41,000
Idaho Falls, Idaho	39,000	26,000	10,000	39,000	—	39,000
Ilion, New York	29,000	13,000	7,000	28,000	1,000	29,000

Urban Area	Population	Fifty Kiloton Bomb (Three Hiroshimas) Killed	Injured	One Megaton Bomb (67 Hiroshimas) Killed	Injured	Twenty Megaton Bomb (1300 Hiroshimas) Killed	Injured
Iowa City, Iowa	54,000	31,000	14,000	53,000	1,000	54,000	—
Ithaca, New York	44,000	30,000	10,000	44,000	—	44,000	—
Jackson, Michigan	80,000	47,000	17,000	76,000	3,000	80,000	—
Jackson, Tennessee	43,000	32,000	7,000	43,000	—	43,000	—
Jacksonville, North Carolina	52,000	16,000	7,000	40,000	10,000	52,000	—
Jacksonville Beach, Florida	52,000	20,000	14,000	48,000	3,000	52,000	—
Jamestown, New York	53,000	33,000	10,000	50,000	2,000	53,000	—
Janesville, Wisconsin	48,000	29,000	12,000	48,000	—	48,000	—
Jefferson City, Missouri	37,000	18,000	11,000	36,000	1,000	37,000	—
Johnson City, Tennessee	43,000	21,000	14,000	43,000	—	43,000	—
Jonesboro, Louisiana	31,000	21,000	5,000	30,000	1,000	31,000	—
Joplin, Missouri	56,000	22,000	15,000	50,000	5,000	56,000	—
Kankakee, Illinois	48,000	24,000	17,000	48,000	—	48,000	—
Kannapolis, North Carolina	76,000	18,000	11,000	55,000	16,000	76,000	—
Key West, Florida	32,000	19,000	9,000	32,000	—	32,000	—
Kingsport, Tennessee	57,000	18,000	16,000	53,000	4,000	57,000	—
Kingston, New York	42,000	23,000	11,000	42,000	—	42,000	—
Kingsville, Texas	28,000	25,000	3,000	28,000	—	28,000	—

Kinston, North Carolina	34,000	28,000	5,000	34,000	—	34,000
Klamath Falls, Oregon	36,000	14,000	10,000	35,000	1,000	36,000
Kokomo, Indiana	64,000	30,000	18,000	61,000	3,000	64,000
La Crosse, Wisconsin	68,000	38,000	12,000	62,000	5,000	68,000
Lafayette, Indiana	80,000	29,000	20,000	78,000	2,000	80,000
Lake Charles, Louisiana	96,000	23,000	31,000	86,000	7,000	96,000
Lancaster, California	33,000	27,000	5,000	33,000	—	33,000
Lancaster, Ohio	40,000	27,000	11,000	40,000	—	40,000
Laredo, Texas	76,000	51,000	16,000	76,000	—	76,000
Las Cruces, Minnesota	59,000	27,000	20,000	58,000	1,000	59,000
Latrobe, Pennsylvania	26,000	14,000	7,000	25,000	1,000	26,000
Laurel, Maryland	49,000	21,000	15,000	48,000	1,000	49,000
Lawrence, Kansas	52,000	30,000	16,000	52,000	—	52,000
Leavenworth, Kansas	38,000	17,000	13,000	36,000	2,000	38,000
Lebanon, Pennsylvania	49,000	31,000	12,000	48,000	1,000	49,000
Lewiston, Idaho	30,000	13,000	8,000	29,000	1,000	30,000
Lewiston, Maine	66,000	39,000	15,000	65,000	1,000	66,000
Lima, Ohio	63,000	33,000	18,000	63,000	—	63,000
Livermore, California	37,000	24,000	9,000	37,000	—	37,000
Lockport, New York	29,000	21,000	6,000	29,000	—	29,000
Lodi, California	31,000	24,000	5,000	31,000	—	31,000
Logan, Vermont	30,000	20,000	7,000	30,000	—	30,000
Longview, Texas	53,000	22,000	14,000	49,000	3,000	53,000
Longview, Washington	51,000	24,000	15,000	51,000	—	51,000
Lynchburg, Virginia	75,000	25,000	24,000	71,000	4,000	75,000

Urban Area	Population	Fifty Kiloton Bomb (Three Hiroshimas)		One Megaton Bomb (67 Hiroshimas)		Twenty Megaton Bomb (1380 Hiroshimas)	
		Killed	Injured	Killed	Injured	Killed	Injured
Manhattan, Kansas	32,000	22,000	9,000	32,000	—	32,000	—
Manitowoc, Wisconsin	32,000	20,000	7,000	32,000	—	32,000	—
Mankato, Minnesota	38,000	26,000	9,000	38,000	—	38,000	—
Mansfield, Ohio	73,000	32,000	23,000	70,000	3,000	73,000	—
Marion, Indiana	42,000	21,000	14,000	42,000	—	42,000	—
Marion, Ohio	45,000	33,000	9,000	45,000	—	45,000	—
Marlborough, Connecticut	26,000	25,000	1,000	26,000	—	26,000	—
Marshalltown, Iowa	27,000	21,000	4,000	27,000	—	27,000	—
Martinsville, Virginia	29,000	14,000	8,000	26,000	3,000	29,000	—
Maryville, Tennessee	36,000	17,000	11,000	36,000	—	36,000	—
Mason City, Iowa	30,000	22,000	8,000	30,000	—	30,000	—
McAllen, Texas	75,000	37,000	14,000	70,000	4,000	75,000	—
Medford, Oregon	41,000	28,000	10,000	41,000	—	41,000	—
Melbourne, Florida	46,000	18,000	7,000	37,000	7,000	46,000	—
Merced, California	36,000	22,000	11,000	36,000	—	36,000	—
Meriden, Connecticut	54,000	35,000	15,000	54,000	—	54,000	—
Meridian, Mississippi	54,000	26,000	18,000	54,000	—	54,000	—
Merritt Island, Florida	63,000	16,000	20,000	57,000	5,000	63,000	—
Michigan City, Indiana	37,000	28,000	7,000	37,000	—	37,000	—
Middletown, Connecticut	41,000	24,000	13,000	41,000	—	41,000	—

Middletown, New York	31,000	22,000	7,000	31,000	—	31,000
Midland, Michigan	38,000	32,000	5,000	38,000	—	38,000
Midland, Texas	64,000	25,000	17,000	62,000	2,000	64,000
Milledgeville, Georgia	26,000	17,000	7,000	26,000	—	26,000
Minot, North Dakota	35,000	23,000	8,000	35,000	—	35,000
Mission Viejo, California	45,000	22,000	16,000	45,000	—	45,000
Missoula, Montana	49,000	26,000	15,000	49,000	—	49,000
Monessen, Pennsylvania	66,000	15,000	20,000	56,000	7,000	66,000
Monroe, Michigan	39,000	26,000	10,000	39,000	—	39,000
Morgantown, West Virginia	40,000	25,000	11,000	40,000	—	40,000
Mundelein, Illinois	36,000	18,000	11,000	36,000	—	36,000
Murfreesboro, Tennessee	32,000	20,000	9,000	32,000	—	32,000
Muskogee, Oklahoma	38,000	23,000	11,000	38,000	—	38,000
Napa, California	57,000	29,000	17,000	56,000	1,000	57,000
Nashua, New Hampshire	68,000	45,000	17,000	68,000	—	68,000
Natchez, Mississippi	33,000	17,000	9,000	32,000	1,000	33,000
Nederland, Texas	33,000	17,000	11,000	33,000	—	33,000
New Castle, Indiana	25,000	21,000	4,000	25,000	—	25,000
New Castle, Pennsylvania	55,000	26,000	18,000	55,000	—	55,000
New Iberia, Louisiana	33,000	22,000	9,000	33,000	—	33,000
New London, Connecticut	57,000	25,000	19,000	55,000	2,000	57,000
New Philadelphia, Ohio	29,000	14,000	9,000	29,000	—	29,000

Urban Area	Population	Fifty Kiloton Bomb (Three Hiroshimas) Killed	Injured	One Megaton Bomb (67 Hiroshimas) Killed	Injured	Twenty Megaton Bomb (1300 Hiroshimas) Killed	Injured
Newark, New Jersey	52,000	29,000	14,000	52,000	—	52,000	—
Newburyport, Massachusetts	26,000	12,000	4,000	24,000	2,000	26,000	—
Newport, Rhode Island	49,000	30,000	13,000	49,000	—	49,000	—
Norman, Oklahoma	61,000	38,000	15,000	61,000	—	61,000	—
Norwich, Connecticut	40,000	25,000	10,000	39,000	1,000	40,000	—
Oak Ridge, Tennessee	28,000	11,000	9,000	28,000	—	28,000	—
Ocala, Florida	49,000	30,000	11,000	48,000	1,000	49,000	—
Oceanside, California	70,000	27,000	22,000	65,000	4,000	70,000	—
Olympia, Washington	53,000	20,000	18,000	49,000	4,000	53,000	—
Orange, New Jersey	33,000	24,000	6,000	33,000	—	33,000	—
Oshkosh, Wisconsin	55,000	41,000	10,000	55,000	—	55,000	—
Ottumwa, Iowa	30,000	15,000	10,000	30,000	—	30,000	—
Owensboro, Kentucky	54,000	33,000	15,000	54,000	—	54,000	—
Paducah, Kentucky	36,000	19,000	10,000	35,000	1,000	36,000	—
Panama City, Florida	48,000	21,000	14,000	45,000	3,000	48,000	—
Parkersburg, West Virginia	65,000	28,000	18,000	59,000	5,000	65,000	—
Pascagoula, Mississippi	60,000	28,000	12,000	58,000	2,000	60,000	—
Pasco, Washington	56,000	18,000	18,000	55,000	1,000	56,000	—
Peekskill, New York	66,000	20,000	13,000	49,000	13,000	66,000	—

Pekin, Illinois	36,000	26,000	7,000	36,000	—	36,000
Peru, Illinois	28,000	17,000	5,000	27,000	1,000	28,000
Petaluma, California	33,000	24,000	7,000	33,000	—	33,000
Pine Bluff, Arkansas	62,000	26,000	20,000	60,000	2,000	62,000
Pittsfield, Massachusetts	62,000	38,000	15,000	60,000	1,000	62,000
Plattsburgh, New York	30,000	20,000	8,000	30,000	—	30,000
Pleasantville, New York	49,000	14,000	10,000	38,000	9,000	49,000
Pocatello, Idaho	45,000	29,000	12,000	45,000	—	45,000
Ponca City, Oklahoma	26,000	19,000	5,000	26,000	—	26,000
Port Arthur, Texas	75,000	24,000	25,000	68,000	5,000	75,000
Port Huron, Michigan	56,000	26,000	16,000	51,000	4,000	56,000
Portsmouth, Virginia	29,000	18,000	8,000	28,000	1,000	29,000
Pottstown, Pennsylvania	35,000	24,000	8,000	35,000	—	35,000
Pottsville, Pennsylvania	38,000	17,000	11,000	37,000	1,000	38,000
Poughkeepsie, New York	58,000	36,000	13,000	56,000	2,000	58,000
Quincy, Illinois	48,000	37,000	9,000	48,000	—	48,000
Rantoul, Illinois	25,000	20,000	5,000	25,000	—	25,000
Rapid City, South Dakota	51,000	24,000	15,000	50,000	1,000	51,000
Redding, California	39,000	14,000	16,000	38,000	1,000	39,000
Redlands, California	48,000	25,000	15,000	48,000	—	48,000
Richland, Washington	33,000	25,000	7,000	33,000	—	33,000
Richmond, Indiana	44,000	28,000	12,000	44,000	—	44,000
Rochester, Minnesota	59,000	36,000	15,000	58,000	1,000	59,000
Rock Hill, South Carolina	43,000	21,000	15,000	43,000	—	43,000

Urban Area	Population	Fifty Kiloton Bomb (Three Hiroshimas) Killed	Injured	One Megaton Bomb (67 Hiroshimas) Killed	Injured	Twenty Megaton Bomb (1300 Hiroshimas) Killed	Injured
Rocky Mount, North Carolina	42,000	25,000	10,000	41,000	1,000	42,000	—
Rome, Georgia	52,000	17,000	18,000	47,000	5,000	52,000	—
Rome, New York	38,000	26,000	10,000	38,000	—	38,000	—
Roswell, New Mexico	41,000	23,000	13,000	41,000	—	41,000	—
Roy, Utah	65,000	14,000	12,000	41,000	17,000	65,000	—
St. Charles, Illinois	59,000	36,000	15,000	59,000	—	59,000	—
St. Cloud, New Mexico	56,000	30,000	18,000	56,000	—	56,000	—
St. Joseph, Missouri	69,000	32,000	17,000	66,000	3,000	69,000	—
Salina, Kansas	39,000	28,000	8,000	39,000	—	39,000	—
Salinas, California	70,000	26,000	23,000	70,000	—	70,000	—
Salisbury, North Carolina	45,000	21,000	13,000	42,000	2,000	45,000	—
San Angelo, Texas	70,000	24,000	27,000	68,000	2,000	70,000	—
San Clemente, California	36,000	19,000	4,000	32,000	3,000	36,000	—
San Luis Obispo, California	38,000	29,000	7,000	38,000	—	38,000	—
Sandusky, Ohio	41,000	27,000	9,000	41,000	—	41,000	—
Sanford, Florida	48,000	36,000	10,000	48,000	1,000	48,000	—
Santa Fe, New Mexico	48,000	27,000	12,000	47,000	—	48,000	—
Santa Maria, California	55,000	28,000	7,000	45,000	8,000	55,000	—
Sedalia, Missouri	25,000	19,000	4,000	25,000	—	25,000	—

Selma, Alabama	31,000	21,000	7,000	31,000	—	31,000	·
Sharon, Pennsylvania	56,000	32,000	17,000	56,000	—	56,000		
Shawnee, Oklahoma	29,000	21,000	6,000	29,000	—	29,000		
Sheboygan, Michigan	52,000	35,000	13,000	52,000	—	52,000		
Sherman, Texas	30,000	22,000	5,000	30,000	—	30,000		
Simi Valley, California	78,000	31,000	22,000	72,000	5,000	78,000		
Sioux Falls, South Dakota	76,000	29,000	30,000	75,000	1,000	76,000		
Southington, Connecticut	27,000	16,000	7,000	27,000	—	27,000	
Spartanburg, South Carolina	77,000	24,000	31,000	75,000	2,000	77,000	
State College, Pennsylvania	41,000	36,000	4,000	41,000	—	41,000	
Statesville, North Carolina	28,000	17,000	8,000	28,000	—	28,000		
Staunton, Virginia	25,000	18,000	5,000	25,000	—	25,000		
Sterling, Illinois	30,000	22,000	6,000	30,000	—	30,000	
Steubenville, Ohio	79,000	23,000	16,000	60,000	15,000	79,000	
Stevens Point, Wisconsin	30,000	24,000	4,000	30,000	—	30,000	
Stillwater, Oklahoma	33,000	24,000	8,000	33,000	—	33,000	
Sumter, South Carolina	43,000	22,000	11,000	43,000	—	43,000		
Taunton, Massachusetts	39,000	24,000	10,000	39,000	—	39,000		
Temple, Texas	43,000	26,000	12,000	43,000	—	43,000		
Terre Haute, Indiana	43,000	18,000	73,000	72,000	—	73,000	

1,000

Urban Area	Population	Fifty Kiloton Bomb (Three Hiroshimas) Killed	Injured	One Megaton Bomb (67 Hiroshimas) Killed	Injured	Twenty Megaton Bomb (1300 Hiroshimas) Killed	Injured
Texarkana, Texas	56,000	27,000	14,000	55,000	1,000	56,000	—
Texas City, Texas	60,000	23,000	11,000	55,000	4,000	60,000	—
Thousand Oaks, California	61,000	26,000	17,000	55,000	4,000	61,000	—
Titusville, Pennsylvania	36,000	12,000	10,000	32,000	4,000	36,000	—
Torrington, Connecticut	29,000	26,000	3,000	29,000	—	29,000	—
Tyler, Texas	65,000	27,000	25,000	64,000	1,000	65,000	—
Uniontown, Pennsylvania	29,000	23,000	5,000	29,000	—	29,000	—
Valdosta, Georgia	39,000	24,000	10,000	39,000	—	39,000	—
Vicksburg, Mississippi	40,000	28,000	10,000	40,000	—	40,000	—
Victoria, Texas	45,000	28,000	11,000	45,000	—	45,000	—
Vineland, New Jersey	42,000	29,000	6,000	42,000	—	42,000	—
Visalia, California	43,000	26,000	12,000	43,000	—	43,000	—
Vista, California	33,000	21,000	8,000	33,000	—	33,000	—
Wahiawa, Hawaii	48,000	22,000	14,000	46,000	2,000	48,000	—
Walla Walla, Washington	34,000	22,000	6,000	33,000	1,000	34,000	—
Wallingford, Connecticut	31,000	24,000	8,000	31,000	—	31,000	—
Warner Robins, Georgia	47,000	24,000	15,000	47,000	—	47,000	—
Washington, Pennsylvania	29,000	23,000	6,000	29,000	—	29,000	—
Watertown, New York	32,000	29,000	2,000	32,000	—	32,000	—

Waterville, Maine	31,000	19,000	8,000	30,000	1,000	31,000
Wausau, Wisconsin	52,000	28,000	11,000	48,000	3,000	52,000
West Chester, Pennsylvania	37,000	27,000	6,000	37,000	—	37,000
West Haverstraw, New York	42,000	24,000	12,000	42,000	—	42,000
West Memphis, Arizona	27,000	18,000	7,000	27,000	—	27,000
Williamsport, Pennsylvania	64,000	26,000	20,000	58,000	5,000	64,000
Wilmington, North Carolina	68,000	33,000	19,000	67,000	1,000	68,000
Wilson, North Carolina	32,000	27,000	4,000	32,000	—	32,000
Winona, Minnesota	29,000	14,000	10,000	29,000	—	29,000
Winter Haven, Florida	59,000	13,000	20,000	52,000	5,000	59,000
Woodbridge, Virginia	62,000	30,000	17,000	61,000	1,000	62,000
Xenia, Ohio	26,000	21,000	5,000	26,000	—	26,000
Yakima, Washington	70,000	31,000	22,000	69,000	1,000	70,000
Yuba City, California	54,000	21,000	11,000	51,000	3,000	54,000
Yuma, Arizona	39,000	17,000	11,000	39,000	—	39,000
Zanesville, Ohio	40,000	20,000	13,000	39,000	1,000	40,000

Damage from a One-Megaton Air Burst at a Height of about 6000 Feet

Peak Wind Velocity (mph)	Peak Pressure (psi)	Distance from Ground Zero	
		Miles	
		11	Light Damage to Window Frames and Doors. Moderate Plaster Damage out to about 15 Miles; Glass Breakage Possible out to 30 Miles
44	1.2		
		10	Second-Degree Burns
		9	
51			Fine Kindling Fuels: Ignited
		8	
60			
		7	
72	2.1		Smokestacks: Slight Damage
		6	30% of Trees Blown Down
98			Wood-Frame Buildings: Moderate Damage. Radio and TV Transmitting Towers: Moderate Damage
		5	Wood-Frame Buildings: Severe Damage Telephone and Power Lines: Limit of Significant Damage
117	3.5		
		4	Third-Degree Burns Wall-Bearing, Brick Buildings (Apartment House Type): Severe Damage
177	5.5		Standard Building Materials Ignite
		3	Light Steel-Frame, Industrial Building: Severe Damage Multistory, Wall-Bearing Buildings (Monumental Type): Severe Damage
278	9.4		
		2	Highway and RR Truss Bridges: Moderate Damage Transportation Vehicles: Moderate Damage
464	18.0		Multistory, Reinforced Concrete Frame Buildings (Office Type): Severe Damage
		1	
307	27.0		
			All (Above Ground) Structures: Severely Damaged or Destroyed
		0	Ground Zero

44

fuel supplies. Intense local fires may combine to produce mass firestorms that will kill large numbers of people in the immediate area, and cremate or asphyxiate even those in blast shelters; in other cases, flames may coalesce into vast, spreading fires called conflagrations, swept along by winds over broad areas.

The second effect of the explosion will be the blast, which kills by generating pressures and winds of almost inconceivable force. The shock wave of the initial blast will explode out from ground zero for miles in all directions, at gradually decreasing levels of intensity. Scientists measure these pressures in units called "psi" (pounds per square inch) and delineate the various levels of pressure resulting from a nuclear explosion by superimposing concentric circles over the map of the target city, with ground zero at the bulls-eye. Similar circles are drawn for the levels of nuclear radiation and thermal effects. Every major city in the United States is probably a bull's-eye in this nuclear target practice by Soviet military planners (and every major city in the Soviet Union is undoubtedly being targeted by American planners). These war planners try to devise nuclear weapon "footprints" for the maximum heat, blast, and radiation damage to cities, industries, and people.

Close to the center of the blast, sudden vast changes in pressure will crush even the most heavily reinforced buildings, much as a beer can is crumpled by a squeeze of the hand. Winds will exceed 160 miles an hour at a distance four miles from ground zero after a one-megaton blast, more than twice the velocity needed to reach hurricane force. The magnitude of the blast effect will depend on the height above ground of the explosion and the distance from ground zero. Soviet planners would use ground level blasts to try to destroy our missiles in hardened silos, and higher altitude blasts to destroy factories, power plants, and other industrial targets over as wide an area as possible. It turns out that human beings in the open are more resistant to the heavy crushing pressure of the blast than to the violent pressure of the wind; four miles from ground zero, a man or woman in the open might survive the blast pressure, only to be picked up, propelled and crushed by killer winds. People in their offices will die in the tangled wreckage as buildings are twisted apart, or they'll be blown out of their skyscrapers if they're "lucky" enough not to be caught in the debris plunging to the streets below.

The third consequence of the explosion is nuclear radiation. Intense doses suffered over six or seven days will kill within a few weeks. Scientists measure radiation dosage to humans in "rem" units: a typical chest X-ray, for example, delivers 0.05 rem to a patient. Ninety percent of those who receive doses of 600 rem in a week—the equivalent of 12,000 chest x-rays—will die; 450 rem will produce 50 percent fatalities; and 300 rem will produce 10 percent fatalities. Fifty to 250 rem will produce nausea and reduce resistance to disease; doses that are not quickly fatal can produce critical long-term effects, such as lethal cancers and leukemias in the victims themselves and genetic deformations in their children. Many scientists feel that any radiation at all is dangerous to some extent over the long term, and that there is no threshold level below which exposure is "safe."

The nuclear radiation peril comes in two stages: intense direct radiation at the time of the blast, within a relatively limited radius; and fallout radiation, created as particles caught up in the blast return to earth. The fallout danger is greatest from a ground level explosion, since tons of irradiated dirt, pulverized buildings, and human flesh are sucked up into the stem and the cap of the mushroom cloud before drifting back to ground. The consequences of exposure to radiation from fallout are similar to those from direct radiation, except that the effects are spread over broader areas defined by the prevailing winds after the blast. Persons suffering high doses will die from radiation sickness; those receiving lighter doses will suffer milder effects and longer-term risks of cancer and genetic disease. The danger decreases over time as the radioactivity in the fallout decays. By current standards of "acceptable" radiation doses, it could be ten years before it is "safe" to return to territory in the first 30 miles of the fallout path. As we have seen already, cancer rates among the Hiroshima survivors soared over the ensuing decades to 5, 15, and 40 times the normal rates. So did mental retardation and chromosome damage.

An additional effect of a nuclear explosion, less threatening to human life but extremely disruptive all the same, is the generation of a massive burst of energy called an electromagnetic pulse, which is somewhat like lightning, but of shorter duration. The pulse is unlikely to kill or injure many human beings, but it can act over vast distances to destroy electrical equipment, power lines, and communications systems; in the case of high-altitude explosions, these effects could travel thousands of miles.

One chilling portion of the OTA study assessed the specific effects of detonating a one-megaton nuclear weapon over the city of Detroit. The attack is assumed to take place without warning, at night when people are at home, and in clear weather. This hypothetical nuclear explosion takes place at ground level, and ground zero is the Renaissance Center in downtown Detroit, where President Reagan stayed during the Republican Convention that nominated him for President in 1980.

The explosion produces a crater three football fields wide and about 70 yards deep. At the edge of the crater is a 200-yard band of highly radioactive debris spewed out of the crater by the blast. Virtually everything is vaporized within a half-mile radius from ground zero, and virtually no buildings remain standing in a 1.7-mile radius. All 70,000 people in this area die instantly; 200,000 die instantly if the blast takes place during working hours.

As far as three miles from ground zero, all homes are totally destroyed; only the foundations and basements are left. The walls of most commercial and apartment buildings are blown out, but their skeletons are left standing; heavy industrial plants may survive at the outer edge of the band. One hundred and thirty thousand people, half of the population in this band, are killed, mostly by collapsing buildings, and almost all of the rest are injured. Up to 5 miles out, more buildings and people survive, but the toll of destruction and injury is still massive. Five percent of the population, or 20,000 people, die immediately and nearly 50 percent, 180,000 people suffer injuries. Fires, which were less of a factor closer to ground zero because essentially all structures were totally destroyed, rage for 24 hours and consume half of the buildings. Finally, in the outer seven miles from ground zero, deaths and damage to physical structures are relatively light, but injury strikes a quarter of the population or 150,000 people.

Because the blast occurs at night, relatively "few" persons, about 8000, die from thermal radiation burns inflicted in the line of sight of the nuclear fireball, and 3000 more are injured. But if the blast occurs instead on a summer weekend afternoon, 190,000 will be burned to death and 75,000 will be injured.

Immediately after the burst, the principal fallout danger comes from the stem of the mushroom cloud. It begins in ten minutes, lasts about an hour, and blankets a six-mile radius. The fallout includes a life-threatening hot spot shaped like an ellipse, moving in the direction of the wind. In an hour, the main fallout from the cap of the cloud itself starts delivering lethal doses of radiation to unprotected persons in its path. Over the next week, with a 15-mph wind from the northwest, the reach of deadly radiation eventually extends past Cleveland all the way to Youngstown, 150 miles away.

This study of Detroit also depicted the consequence of this ground burst if the same size weapon explodes 6000 feet in the air. Twice as many people are killed by the air burst, many thousands are injured, and the bands for blast damage, thermal burns, and fires increase about 25 percent in width. There is no crater, and reinforced buildings near ground zero are left part intact.

Finally, the study examined the effects of a 25 megaton explosion on Detroit. Even larger numbers of people are killed and wounded; virtually the entire metropolitan area is destroyed or heavily damaged. The study concludes that "rescue operations will have to be totally supported from outside the area, with the evacuation of survivors the only feasible course. Recovery and rebuilding will be a very long-term problematical issue." But what if other cities are under simultaneous attack, there is no outside help, and there is no refuge for the refugees?

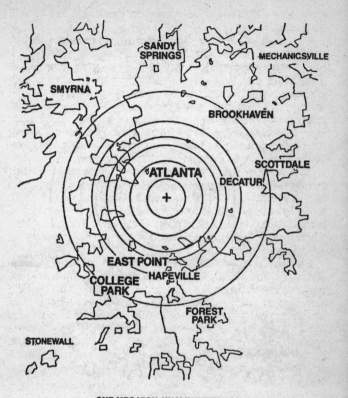

ONE-MEGATON NUCLEAR WEAPON
Air Burst

Circle   Effects

6. 2 psi: Houses moderately damaged
5. 12 cal/cm²: Third-degree burns
4. 25 cal/cm²: Spontaneous ignition
3. 5 psi: Houses destroyed
2. 10 psi: Masonry buildings destroyed
1. 20 psi: Reinforced concrete buildings destroyed
+ "Ground Zero"

Atlanta, Georgia county lines

49

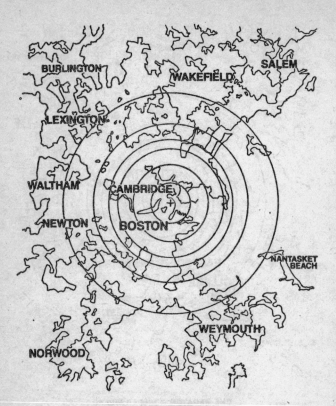

ONE-MEGATON NUCLEAR WEAPON
Air Burst

Circle   Effects

6. 2 psi: Houses moderately damaged
5. 12 cal/cm³: Third-degree burns
4. 25 cal/cm³: Spontaneous ignition
3. 5 psi: Houses destroyed
2. 10 psi: Masonry buildings destroyed
1. 20 psi: Reinforced concrete buildings destroyed
+ "Ground Zero"

Boston, Massachusetts county lines

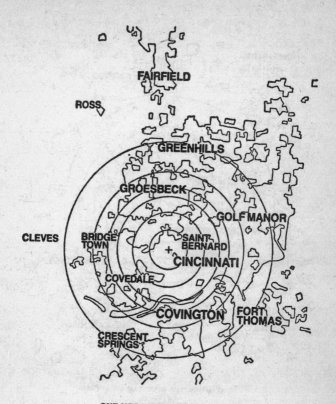

ONE-MEGATON NUCLEAR WEAPON
Air Burst

Circle   Effects

6. 2 psi: Houses moderately damaged
5. 12 cal/cm²: Third-degree burns
4. 25 cal/cm²: Spontaneous ignition
3. 5 psi: Houses destroyed
2. 10 psi: Masonry buildings destroyed
1. 20 psi: Reinforced concrete buildings destroyed
+ "Ground Zero"

Cincinnati, Ohio, and Covington, Kentucky county lines

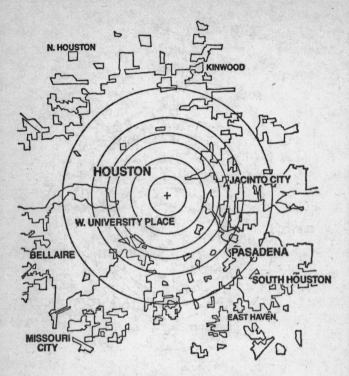

ONE-MEGATON NUCLEAR WEAPON
Air Burst

Circle   Effects

6. 2 psi: Houses moderately damaged
5. 12 cal/cm³: Third-degree burns
4. 25 cal/cm³: Spontaneous ignition
3. 5 psi: Houses destroyed
2. 10 psi: Masonry buildings destroyed
1. 20 psi: Reinforced concrete buildings destroyed
+ "Ground Zero"

Houston, Texas county lines

52

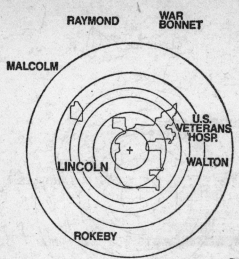

RAYMOND   WAR BONNET

MALCOLM

U.S. VETERANS HOSP.

LINCOLN   WALTON

ROKEBY

BENNET

HANLON SIDING

ONE-MEGATON NUCLEAR WEAPON
Air Burst

Circle   Effects

6. 2 psi: Houses moderately damaged
5. 12 cal/cm²: Third-degree burns
4. 25 cal/cm²: Spontaneous ignition
3. 5 psi: Houses destroyed
2. 10 psi: Masonry buildings destroyed
1. 20 psi: Reinforced concrete buildings destroyed
+ "Ground Zero"

Lincoln, Nebraska county lines

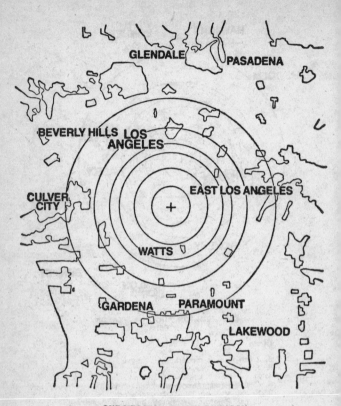

ONE-MEGATON NUCLEAR WEAPON
Air Burst

Circle   Effects

6. 2 psi: Houses moderately damaged
5. 12 cal/cm²: Third-degree burns
4. 25 cal/cm²: Spontaneous ignition
3. 5 psi: Houses destroyed
2. 10 psi: Masonry buildings destroyed
1. 20 psi: Reinforced concrete buildings destroyed
+ "Ground Zero"

Los Angeles, California county lines

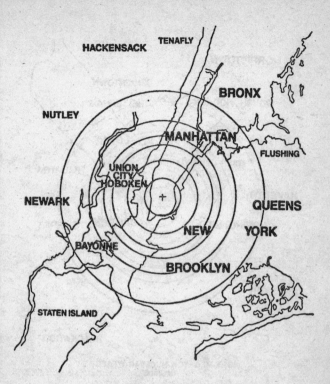

ONE-MEGATON NUCLEAR WEAPON
Air Burst

Circle   Effects

6. 2 psi: Houses moderately damaged
5. 12 cal/cm³: Third-degree burns
4. 25 cal/cm³: Spontaneous ignition
3. 5 psi: Houses destroyed
2. 10 psi: Masonry buildings destroyed
1. 20 psi: Reinforced concrete buildings destroyed
+ "Ground Zero"

New York, New York county lines

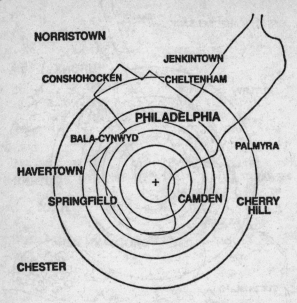

ONE-MEGATON NUCLEAR WEAPON
Air Burst

Circle   Effects

6. 2 psi: Houses moderately damaged
5. 12 cal/cm²: Third-degree burns
4. 25 cal/cm³: Spontaneous ignition
3. 5 psi: Houses destroyed
2. 10 psi: Masonry buildings destroyed
1. 20 psi: Reinforced concrete buildings destroyed
+ "Ground Zero"

Philadelphia, Pennsylvania county lines

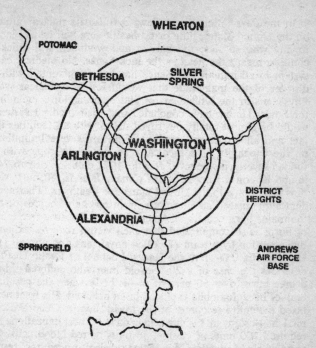

ONE-MEGATON NUCLEAR WEAPON
Air Burst

Circle   Effects

6. 2 psi: Houses moderately damaged
5. 12 cal/cm²: Third-degree burns
4. 25 cal/cm²: Spontaneous ignition
3. 5 psi: Houses destroyed
2. 10 psi: Masonry buildings destroyed
1. 20 psi: Reinforced concrete buildings destroyed
+ "Ground Zero"

Washington, DC county lines

In the devastation that follows a full-scale nuclear attack on the United States, little or no health care will be available to any who survive; the burned and wounded will quickly come to regard the dead as the lucky ones. No medical care system in all human experience has been confronted with a disaster of the magnitude that would follow a nuclear war. Physicians in the United States and other nations, including the Soviet Union, have concluded that their medical systems would be almost totally destroyed. Even with all facilities intact and all physicians on duty, there are severe limitations on the capability of a medical care system to cope with a sudden severe emergency. After the 1977 collision of two 747 jumbo jets on a runway in the Canary Islands, 50 burn victims were flown to the United States for treatment. That accident alone placed an enormous strain on the resources of all the major burn centers in America. Why? Because treatment of burns is so complicated that each victim requires exhaustive attention by a team of skilled physicians and nurses. Dr. Howard Hiatt, Dean of the Harvard School of Public Health, describes the case of a 20-year-old man who suffered third-degree burns over 90 percent of his body when the gasoline tank of his automobile exploded in an accident. His treatment taxed the entire resources of the Massachusetts General Hospital in Boston; in the first eight days of hospitalization, he required 100 units of plasma, 40 units of red blood cells, 12 units of blood platelets, five major surgical procedures, respirator care, and round-the-clock specialized nursing.

In 1981, the extraordinary emergency care provided by George Washington University Hospital in Washington, D.C., saved the lives of President Reagan and his press secretary, James Brady. Fifty victims with similar injuries arriving in the emergency room at the same time would have definitely overloaded the capacity of that hospital for effective treatment. A few hundred patients with the same injuries would have overloaded all the hospitals in the city. Now consider a 6000-megaton attack on the United States which the Federal Emergency Management Agency, assigned the task of planning for nuclear disaster, calls a model CRP-2B attack. It would rain the equivalent of 400,000 Hiroshimas on the nation: the targets would be military installations, industrial facilities, and population centers with 50,000 people or more. Minutes after such an attack, 40 percent of the nation's population—86 million Americans—would be dead; 34 million more would be severely injured, requiring sophisticated emergency care. Within a few weeks at most over half of them would die, most without receiving any medical care at all.

An even higher proportion of all the physicians in the country would be killed—80 percent—since most of them reside and practice in urban areas. Most of the hospitals would also be destroyed. According to this war-game analysis, the 79,000 physicians who survived the attack would have 32 million patients to treat: 18 million suffering from radiation sickness and 14 million suffering from severe trauma or burns. As Dr. Geiger testified in 1980, the survivors would have "ruptured lungs, ruptured internal organs, ruptured ear drums, crushed skulls and bodies, penetrating wounds of the skull and chest and abdomen, every conceivable kind of trauma." For these victims there would be little hope, little relief, and little care before they died. On the average, each physician who survived, whether trained as an internist, brain surgeon, psychiatrist, dermatologist, radiologist, or general practitioner, would become, in effect, the entire medical resource for 170 acutely injured patients. Instead of several doctors for each badly burned patient, there would be scores of burned patients for each doctor. Instead of special facilities for treating patients, there would be virtually no facilities and no treatment at all.

The hopelessness of medical help can be illustrated in another way. If each severely injured victim of a nuclear attack on Washington, D.C. required only one-tenth as many units of blood as the auto victim previously mentioned, the city would need 12 million units. The total blood available in the American Red Cross Northeast Stockpile on an average day is 11,000 units; in all of 1979, the total amount of blood donated in the entire United States was 14 million units.

Describing the hypothetical explosion of a single 20-megaton warhead on Boston, Dr. Geiger said:

> We figured in Boston a number of years ago that perhaps 1,600 out of 6,000 physicians would be surviving and functioning at all, creating a ratio perhaps of one physician to every 1,700 injured surviving. And that does not account for or include all the rest of the population with pre-existing dis-

ease, nor for panic, nor for some of the other kinds of phenomena. If every such physician saw each patient with those complex injuries for only 15 minutes and worked for 16 hours a day, it would be from 16 to 26 days before everybody injured would be seen. And most would have died by then. The blunt reality is that most of the injured survivors of any of these specified attacks will die without any medical attention, without even receiving narcotics for their pain, and that in effect the survivors will envy the dead. Further, for physicians to do any of the kinds of things we are talking about—to treat trauma, to separate the seriously injured from the less seriously injured, to separate the lethally radiated from the less radiated—requires, of course, hospitals and complex equipment. They too are concentrated in the areas of highest lethality. And at least 60 percent of all the hospital beds in each of these metropolitan areas, perhaps a higher percentage of the tertiary care beds, would be destroyed even by a one-megaton attack. Now, to this scattering of medical resources and physicians, let us add that there would be no transportation systems, no communication systems, no electric power in most places, no X-rays, no water. Bridges and tunnels have collapsed. What is left of the buildings is lying in what is left of the streets, and both are unrecognizable. The problem of medical care becomes a metaphor for the general problem of both short and long term consequences of this kind of attack; that is, it becomes clear that it makes no sense to talk in terms of physical or biological survival. Human existence is social existence. Medical care is simply one example of a complex social enterprise that would be impossible under these circumstances.

For those who survive the initial blast and do not die from their wounds or burns, more horrors lie ahead. Analyzing the hypothetical 6000-megaton attack cited earlier, Dr. Herbert Abrams of Harvard Medical School summarized the immediate injuries and the ensuing infections and disease:

Medical Problem (in Chronological Order of Occurrence)	Barrage Period	Shelter Period	Early Survival Period
	First Hour	First Day	First Four Weeks	
Flash burns	+			
Trauma and blast injury	+			
Flame burns and smoke inhalation	+	+		
Acute radiation	+			
Fallout radiation	+	+	+	+
Suffocation and heat prostration		+	+	
General lack of medical care		+	+	+
Dehydration			+	
Communicable diseases			+	+
Exposure and hardship			+	+
Malnutrition			+	+
Cancer				
Genetic damage				

Radiation will make the survivors far more vulnerable to infection. As many as 23 million persons may suffer actual radiation sickness, and a comparable number will receive doses of radiation sufficient to decrease their resistance to disease. Many victims with severe burns will die from infection. The absence of adequate food and water will lead to malnutrition and dehydration, which in turn will substantially increase the risk of infection. Inadequate sanitation in mass shelters will accelerate the spread of infection. Insects breeding in unburied bodies of people and animals will become carriers of typhus, malaria, dengue fever, plague, encephalitis, and other crippling diseases; there will be no vaccines available to prevent them and no antibiotics to cure them. Dr. Abrams divided the epidemics most likely to run rampant into two groups:

Epidemics of Diseases Currently of Low Incidence	Epidemics of Serious Existing Diseases
Cholera	Diarrhea
Malaria	Diphtheria
Plague	Hepatitis
Shigellosis	Influenza
Smallpox	Meningitis
Typhoid fever	Pneumonia
Typhus	Tuberculosis
Yellow fever	Whooping cough

In the nineteenth century, tuberculosis was a fearful mass killer, at one time striking down as many as 550 persons for each 100,000 people in New York City. Improvements in housing, fuel, food, sanitation, and drug treatment brought it under control but could not eradicate it. Whenever these improvements are removed, the disease returns; tuberculosis is all around us, merely waiting for the right conditions to flare up, as it did in Warsaw in World War I, in Berlin in World War II, and in Nazi concentration camps. A nuclear attack would unleash a tuberculosis epidemic on the United States whose effects would be even more lethal than similar epidemics in the past; so few are exposed to tuberculosis today that there is little resistance in the population. Other ancient scourges of humanity would also be revived.

Plague, regarded as a disease of the Middle Ages because of the devastating epidemics that swept across Europe in those years, has killed over 12 million people in this century; it is still transmitted today by wild rodents in 11 western states. A nuclear war could suddenly create an ideal environment for its massive spread. It is estimated that 12 percent of all survivors would be infected by plague and half would die from it. Overall, a quarter of those who survived the immediate effects of a nuclear war would probably die from tuberculosis, plague, or other epidemic diseases. Doctors despair of treating either the overwhelming immediate trauma or the longer-term but still lethal consequences of nuclear war. They understand that the public has come to expect miracles of modern medicine to be performed when they are needed, but doctors know that no miracles will be performed on the day of nuclear judgment. That is why so many doctors have joined Physicians for Social Responsibility in order to educate the public to the impossibility of practicing their profession after nuclear war begins. It is also why they support a nuclear weapons freeze; as physicians, they know that where treatment of a disease is hopeless, the only hope is prevention of the disease.

The enormous casualties suffered in a nuclear attack, the instant collapse of the health care system, and the vast destruction of virtually all industrial facilities in the United States is almost impossible for the human mind to conceive. The OTA study referred to earlier in this chapter sought to make its own assessment of the consequences of an all-out nuclear war with thousands of Soviet warheads exploding across the United States, simultaneously creating hundreds of thousands of Hiroshimas. One hundred and sixty-five million Americans could be killed in such an attack, or two-thirds of the population of the nation. The study concluded: "[T]he number of deaths and the damage and destruction inflicted on the U.S. society and economy by the sheer magnitude of such an attack would place in question whether the United States would ever recover its position as an organized, industrial, and powerful country." The death of Detroit, for example, would result from a single nuclear burst; all-out nuclear war would mean the economic, political, and social death, and perhaps even the physical death, of the entire United States.

Finally, the OTA report imagined the impact of an all-out nuclear war on a city not directly hit: Charlottesville, Virginia. The nearest targets of Soviet attack would be Washington and Richmond; Charlottesville would escape the initial holocaust. But given the extent of the destruction in the rest of the nation, the city would become a falling domino of nuclear war. Its life and structure would disintegrate as refugees suffering from radiation sickness poured in. Hospitals would fill their beds and then lock their doors. Squatters willing to risk the lingering fallout would seize the homes of those still living in fallout shelters. To ward off anarchy, an emergency local government would have to be created and an informal martial law declared. Eventually, people in Charlottesville would hear that a 4000-megaton Soviet attack on U.S. military and industrial targets had killed over one hundred million people. The Northeast Corridor from Boston to Norfolk would be a "swath of burning rubble."

A cease-fire would probably be put in place, but it would be a freeze too late. Both the United States and the Soviet Union would retain enough nuclear power to dissuade other nations from attacking or invading their stricken lands. Dreamers would talk of rebuilding the United States on the time scale of the German and Japanese recoveries from the previous world war, but realists would recognize that there was no longer prosperity in America to offer a helping hand. Others would speak of models for a postnuclear American society based on the struggling economies of the poorest nations of Asia or Latin America.

The President and a remnant of Congress would be attempting to function in the rural Midwest, with Congress ceding absolute powers to the President. But few links would be established between Charlottesville and the new national capital. The federal government would conscript able-bodied young men and women to rebuild areas of devastation, but no records would be available and those who volunteered for the task would be so disillusioned that they would desert and return to Charlottesville.

In subsequent weeks fears would abate and threats of anarchy would subside as the community regrouped, rediscovered agriculture, and revived forgotten cottage industries in a battle for survival. At a conference called at the University of Virginia to contemplate the future, a historian would explain: "We are in the classic race. We have to be able to produce new goods and materials before we exhaust our stored supplies. We can continue to eat the wheat that is in the grain elevators of the Midwest for another year, perhaps. But after that, we have to have the capacity to grow new wheat. When our winter coats wear through, we have to have the capacity to weave the cloth for new ones. When our railroad cars break down, we have to be able to make new ones or replacement parts. Right now, we are a long way from that capacity." Others would argue that technology itself was likely to disappear: "After a while, in a few generations, no one remembers how the machines worked at all. They remember the important things: how to plant crops, how to train horses and oxens, how to make a simple pump. We will have survived biologically, but our way of life is going to be unrecognizable. In several generations, the United States is going to resemble a late medieval society."

That is a possible scenario of a 4000-megaton Soviet attack on American industrial and military targets. The reality could be more megatons and much worse. What if the Soviets have targeted all the Charlottesvilles as well? What if fallout pollutes the soil where the survivors live, and their rations of grain and milk contain dangerous doses of strotium 90, as seems almost certain? The genetic consequences are ominous and unpredictable.

After it happened, the stockpiles of nuclear weaponry would finally be reduced, not because a peaceful agreement had been negotiated, but because they had been used up in war. The nuclear threat sets before us a basic choice. The question is not whether nuclear weapons will cease multiplying and then be reduced. Someday they almost surely will be. The choice is how we will stop the arms race and how we will reduce its arsenals: by rational agreement, or by the most irrational act of violence in human history. This is why it is so very important for each of us to know what will happen if a nuclear war ever comes: each of us must work harder now to prevent it from happening. To see the risk in human terms in our own cities and neighborhoods, to understand what it will do to individual Americans as well as to all of America is an irresistible summons for individuals to take a stand. The only sane choice is to continue the peaceful battle for a nuclear freeze until it is won.

3

THE NEXT NUCLEAR WAR
A WOUNDED WORLD

"No arts; no letters; no society . . . and the
life of man, solitary, poor, nasty, brutish, and
short."

—Thomas Hobbes, 1651

An all-out Soviet nuclear attack against the United States
would precipitate massive retaliation by American nuclear
forces against the Soviet Union. The entire northern hemisphere would be engulfed by this nuclear exchange, and its
effects would slowly spread across the globe.

Officials in the Reagan administration have loosely suggested that nuclear war is "survivable." As evidence they point to
the continued growth of the Soviet Union after the enormous
casualties suffered during World War II, and the rebuilding of
Dresden, Hiroshima, and Nagasaki in the wake of unprecedented destruction in that war. These successes, they claim, il-
lustrate man's capacity to endure and recover. We are to be
reassured, then, that nuclear war, no matter how large in
scale, would merely present another challenge to human
courage, imagination, and spirit.

But such historical analogies and visions of reconstruction
reflect ignorance or deliberate distortion. No previous war,
no volcano, no earthquake, no plague has ever posed the type of
threat to our civilization and our planet as does a general nuclear war.

Jonathan Schell has prophesied that America would become "a republic of insects and grass." To that, some critics and officials of the Reagan administration have responded with the small consolation that the "death of the earth" as a consequence of nuclear conflict is something of an exaggeration. But in reality, and at minimum, the result would be the death of Western and Soviet society. In addition, such a conflict could mean the sickness, perhaps even unto ultimate death, of the whole world. The probability that this outcome—a world down to the last human being—may be low does not highly recommend taking the gamble.

President Reagan is probably right about one thing: after the initial blasts, some human life would be left somewhere. At least initially, some Americans and Soviets, and other human beings, will undoubtedly manage to escape falling buildings, blast effects, charring heat, and massive doses of radiation. But then what will they face? What will become of Earth after an all-out nuclear exchange between the Soviet Union and the United States?

We cannot definitely say. This type of inquiry is, by definition, speculative. We do know, however, that nuclear weapons present a threat to every facet of human existence. For it is not only clear that there will be immediate and incredible casualties and destruction, but that the very foundation of global society will be shaken and the environment so irreversibly altered as to conceivably snuff out human life over time. The two superpowers together have strategic arsenals equivalent to four tons of TNT for every man, woman, and child presently living on this planet. Today, no matter what the optimists about nuclear war may say, the earth itself is an endangered species.

The world's ecosystem is so delicately balanced and intertwined that the effects of a nuclear exchange could not be contained to the United States, the Soviet Union, Europe, or even the northern hemisphere. There would be three grave global effects of a nuclear war: delayed radioactive fallout; dramatic changes in climate; and depletion of the ozone layer. It is the synergy of these effects—the way they interact to produce further effects—that raises the question of whether the earth would be at all habitable after a nuclear war.

When a nuclear bomb explodes, it releases hundreds of types of radioactive isotopes. Dr. Jack Geiger, of City Col-

lege of New York, has reported: "In an exchange, which is a
very realistic possibility, that involves simply 5,000 megatons
on each side, the recent calculations by physicists at Massachusetts Institute of Technology were that there would be five
million square miles of lethal radiation. This is an area the
size of the United States." And that radioactive fallout would
hang in the atmosphere, and move across the seas on shifting
winds. Some of its fission products would be short-lived,
while others would take literally millions of years to decay.
These particles, carried up into the many mushroom clouds
spawned in a large attack and then distributed in the upper
atmosphere circling the globe, would eventually be dispersed
worldwide, not only by rain, but by gravity.

Radioactive contamination spreading around the globe can
have a devastating impact on animal and plant life everywhere, killing millions in every species, breeding mutations
that will reshape the ecosystem, and salting the ground with
poisons that render it permanently fallow. Fallout that does
not reach high enough concentrations to prove immediately
fatal for human beings will lead to radiation sickness, de-
creased resistance to disease, increased rates of cancer of all
types, and genetic defects in succeeding generations. As Albert Einstein warned a generation ago, "Radioactive poisoning of the atmosphere and annihilation of any life on earth
has been brought within the range of technical possibilities."

After wind and rain have carried radioactivity to the
far corners of human existence, its by-products will be ab-
sorbed into the food chains. Contaminated water will feed
plant life which, in turn, will be consumed by animals of all
sorts. To complicate matters, for long periods after the attack,
people will not have the means to determine which supplies
of food and water are safe. It will be nearly impossible to
avoid continued exposure to dangerous amounts of radioactive contamination. Survivors will witness the revival of the
bubonic plague and other pestilence. These constant compan-
ions in the Middle Ages are largely controlled today, but only
held in abeyance by modern sanitation and medical care. Ion-
izing radiation would so weaken resistance to disease that epidemics in crops and animals could rage on a global scale.
Diseased crops and livestock could mean mass starvation in
both the northern and southern hemispheres. Furthermore,
the depletion of food production in "developed" nations

would subtly extend the consequences of nuclear war to the dependent populations of "less developed" nations.

Fallout is only one of many traumatic assaults on nature from such a war. Large numbers of high-yield nuclear weapons will produce up to fifty times the amount of nitrous oxide normally present in the atmosphere. If trillions upon trillions of nitrous oxide molecules swarm into the stratosphere, they can react with ozone to form nitrogen and oxygen by-products. These by-products would deplete the protective ozone layer which, by intercepting most of the ultraviolet rays of the sun, is one of the key environmental factors making life on earth possible.

According to a 1975 study conducted by the National Academy of Sciences (NAS), which posited a 10,000-megaton exchange between the Soviet Union and the United States, "Ozone reductions in the range of 30 to 70 percent are possible." The envisioned attack would be major but not total, and would target only the northern hemisphere. While it is difficult to determine the precise effects of rapid ozone depletion, the incidence of skin cancer would rise dramatically, retinal damage and blinding of animals and humans would rage everywhere, and the increased ultraviolet radiation would contribute to disease on a broad spectrum in both the animal and plant kingdoms. If upper levels of ozone depletion are realized, irreversible injury to ocean species might occur in the years following the detonations. The increased ultraviolet radiation might raise the levels of vitamin D in the skin of mammals and birds to toxic levels.

It is important to recognize, when considering the potential environmental effects of a nuclear war, that the precious ozone layer surrounding our planet is one of the preconditions for most life forms. They have been protected and nurtured under the ozone shield for millions of years. We cannot know with certainty that enough ozone would still be present to prevent the disappearance of human life from the earth. The National Academy of Sciences guessed there would be enough. However, even Dr. Fred Ikle, now Under Secretary of Defense, concedes that ozone depletion due to nuclear war could "shatter the ecological structure that permits man to remain alive on this planet."

The enormous explosive power released by the equivalent of many millions of tons of TNT would also spew huge

amounts of dirt, dust, and ash into the atmosphere, much of
it containing the fine particles and fragments of our society,
the pulverized buildings and the vaporized human beings. In
the short term, much of the northern hemisphere will look
like the area around Mount St. Helens in the aftermath of
volcanic eruption. The sky will darken, and the land will be
covered with a layer of granular, radioactive debris.

In the long term, the soot in the sky could block the heat
of the sun and cause a cooling of the earth, perhaps only by
a few degrees. Even a drop in temperature of two degrees
centigrade could bring the American Midwest a climate like
Canada's. And the possibility of dramatic changes in temperature and weather profiles is very real, particularly because
the dust and the ozone depletion together would batter cli-
matic patterns. The effects might not be uniform, and there
could be a dramatic series of climate reversals. According to
the NAS study of the impact of nuclear war, the synergy of
the dust and ozone effects could be disastrous:

> Climatologists are aware of the possibility that the
> processes that generate world climate and weather
> may be subject to major instabilities and that the
> perturbation of atmospheric conditions and dynam-
> ics might trigger a much larger process and thereby
> initiate a major change in climate.

The potential radical shortening of growing seasons and the
freezing of lakes and rivers, perhaps followed by a sudden
warming trend, could irretrievably change the face of the
earth as we know it today. The polar ice caps might expand
or contract, or undergo both effects in succession, at some
point inundating coastal areas. Today's hills could be the
beachfront of the postnuclear war period.

In addition to enormous uncertainty about human survival
due to the depletion of the ozone and the pollution of the
skies, there are other global assaults on the environment
which we cannot rule out. The destruction of vegetation by
fire, blast, disease, and radiation, for instance, presents an
awesome array of complications. First, these conditions could
contribute to the cooling of the planet, because newly barren
ground would absorb and retain less heat. Second, erosion of
the soil formerly protected by plant life could increase the
mineral content of run-off water, robbing the remaining soil

of nutrients. Increases in algae and microscopic organisms in rivers and streams would deplete oxygen in the water and kill fish and other marine life, while the ground would no longer support any vegetation except perhaps grass.

In the face of the environmental calamities that could result from a major nuclear exchange, it is clear that such a conflict between the Soviet Union and the United States would do far more than kill untold numbers of people. The delicate balance of nature knows no national boundaries. The contamination of food supplies, the spread of disease, the alteration of the earth's climate, and the depletion of the ozone layer may, in sum, catastrophically touch every political power bloc and every part of the earth. Human life, all of human life, might not survive on a progressively hostile planet. Nuclear war could mean evolution in reverse.

The biological and ecological implications of a major nuclear exchange challenge our capacity to predict the dimensions of the disaster. But the effects on our social and political structure, on civilization itself, are no less staggering. The physically and psychologically scarred in both the United States and the Soviet Union who are unfortunate enough to survive an all-out nuclear war will face the Sisyphean task of rebuilding a society out of its shattered shards. In the myth of Sisyphus, the Greek gods condemned him to the perpetual torment of futile labor. His eternal task was to roll a huge stone to the top of a mountain, only to have it roll back down again each time it neared the top. After a nuclear war, the survivors would have to roll countless pebbles and pieces of rubble up a mountain and put them all together again—a job that could require centuries, if it could ever be completed at all.

Life in both America and Russia would likely descend into anarchy or into a hard authoritarianism without even the pretext of concern for individual welfare. Indeed, the economic and political values that have pitted capitalism and communism against each other would become meaningless luxuries in the social dissolution after a nuclear war. As John Kenneth Galbraith has observed:

> . . . If there is a nuclear exchange, large or as some now imagine limited—what is called free enterprise or capitalism will not survive. Nor will free institutions. All will be shattered beyond recovery.

So, equally, will be what is now called communism. Capitalism, communism and socialism are all so-phisticated social forms relevant only to the advanced world as it has now developed. None would have existence or relevance in the wreckage and ashes and among the exiguous survivors of a post-nuclear world. There is no matter of easy rhetoric; involved are hard facts which no one after serious thought can escape.

Those who survived the conflict in both countries would be forced to hunt for food, to ration scarce medical help, and to fight for shelter in a highly radioactive and war-ravaged environment. Starvation would stalk all but the most powerful who could take from others. How would society cope with the new and continuing outbreaks of thyphus, typhoid and cholera? Diabetics would simply die, since it would be at least decades before limited resources could provide enough insulin. Cockroaches and other insects might thrive, but people would have to live like moles in the ground, and even when they emerged, they would confront the prospect of a slow poisoning for generations. In the wake of the war itself, the sick and the injured, sealed indefinitely in the underground confines of their shelters, would be forced to look after themselves.

American society is organized around a system of incentives and monetary rewards that motivate people to produce goods and services for the general well-being. In a world replete with radioactive fallout and debris, there would be little incentive to work toward goals beyond what was necessary for individual or local survival, especially if any effort at all meant risking sickness or death. There would be no reason to venture from relative safety into contaminated areas. This would mean, among other things, that transportation systems would disintegrate, and if there were outsiders somewhere willing to help, there would be no way to move food and medicine to blighted places. Given the difficulty and danger of producing food, it is unlikely that people would struggle to produce it for others, since they would have barely enough for themselves. The primary struggle would be for bare existence, for a rough social organization, and perhaps for dominion over others.

If the survivors looked for aid to nations beyond the immediate battleground, they would find an entire world desperately in need of aid. After a nuclear war, North America, which is the "world's breadbasket," would no longer be providing essential food for Third World countries. The National Academy of Sciences has reported: "Patently, were the U.S. and Canada involved [in nuclear war], these crops would be unavailable for indefinite periods . . . and the death toll due to starvation would rise accordingly."

Even if there were no fallout, and even if civil defense could protect many millions, what would the survivors return to? As much as 80 to 90 percent of America's industrial capacity would be gone, and buildings everywhere would be in ruins. Economic recovery, as the Office of Technology Assessment (OTA) noted, might well be impossible: "It cannot be said whether the productive facilities that physically survived [undamaged or repairable with available supplies and skills] would be adequate to sustain recovery. . . . In effect, the country would enter a race, with economic viability as the prize. The country would try to restore production to the point where consumption of stocks and the wearing out of surviving goods and tools was matched by new production. If this was achieved before stocks ran out, then viability would be attained. Otherwise, consumption would necessarily sink to the level of new production and in so doing would probably depress production further, creating a downward spiral. At some point this spiral would stop, but by the time it did so the United States might have returned to the economic equivalent of the Middle Ages."

Much the same applies to the Soviet industrial infrastructure. As the OTA study says, "There is no evidence that the Soviet economy and its supporting industry would be less severely damaged than their U.S. counterparts. Nor is there any evidence that the Soviets face a lower risk of finding themselves unable to rebuild an industrial society at all."

The OTA study also emphasizes that the unpredictable effects of a nuclear war could enormously magnify the problem of postwar recovery: "The question of how rapid and efficient economic recovery would be—or indeed whether a genuine recovery would be possible at all—raises questions that seem to be beyond calculation. It is possible to calculate direct economic damage by making assumptions about the size and exact location of bomb explosions; however, such calculations cannot address the issues of bottlenecks and of synergy. Bottlenecks would occur if a key product that was essential for many other manufacturing processes could no longer be produced, or [for the case of a large attack] if an entire industrial sector were wiped out. In either case, the economic loss would greatly exceed the peacetime value of the factories that were actually destroyed . . . Apart from the creation of bottlenecks, there could be synergistic effects: for example, the fire that cannot be controlled because the fire destroyed fire stations, as actually happened in Hiroshima. . . . Housing, defined as a place where a productive worker lives as distinct from shelter for refugees, is another area of uncertainty. Minimal housing is essential if production is to be restored, and it takes time to rebuild it if the existing housing stock is destroyed or is beyond commuting range of the surviving [or repaired] workplaces."

Much of the world's expertise in agriculture and technology would perish in nuclear war. The industrial nations contain most of the knowledge and research and development experience upon which the rest of the world depends. The war would destroy not only the United States and the Soviet Union, but almost certainly Europe, the Middle East, and Japan as well. The countries spared direct attack would be cut off from the major sources of applied learning and, whatever else happened, would have vast difficulty recreating or maintaining the advanced technologies we have today. As the National Academy of Sciences has concluded,

> For many nations not directly involved in the hypothesized exchange, their technical capabilities rest in significant measure on the apparatus, equipment, and technicians which would suddenly become unavailable . . . Survivors from affected countries would [also] probably lack the ability to care for themselves, e.g., to monitor fallout, to provide medical care, food and water, or to contain epidemic disease, much less to assist the "less developed" nations in such activities.

More generally, civilization has arrived where it is today by using up the cheaper and more accessible resources, and gradually learning to fathom the more difficult ones. How could survivors struggle back to the civilization we know today when the easy sources, such as forests, wild animals, and shallow oil reserves, have already been thoroughly exploited?

One can imagine part of our population surviving, but they would be living in an anomalous situation more suited to the Dark Ages. Individuals would be driven by the goal of self-sufficiency. They would be tied to the land, and there would be little or no manufacturing on a mass scale. Force would probably become the means by which the surviving society would motivate people to work. As General George Seignious, former Director of the U.S. Arms Control and Disarmament Agency, has written, "Nuclear war would as surely destroy our freedom as Soviet tanks upon our streets."

Those who think of nuclear war as a way of defending freedom or Western values are living in the past. In John Kenneth Galbraith's words, "Those who say we must accept the risk of nuclear conflict to save our system are saying, in the strongest possible terms, that we should accept its certain destruction. . . . We must not, regardless of politics, continue to imagine that we can protect or save an economic system, by accepting the possibility of nuclear war. In the ashes, communism and capitalism, let it be said again, will be indistinguishable. They will also be indistinguishable and irrelevant in the ultra-primitive struggle for existence for those who are unfortunate enough to survive."

And those survivors would find themselves a different, deeper, and darker age than the one which descended on Europe fifteen hundred years ago. Then the oldest centers of Western civilization, although damaged, also endured. When human beings began to see through the darkness, they looked for light and for the recovery of collective memory to Rome, Athens, and vast manuscript collections in monasteries across the continent. Much of ancient art and sculpture was recovered. The Renaissance did not recreate the human heritage, but reawakened to it. This time, when men and women in the northern hemisphere, if they win the struggle for survival at all, look for the light of the past, where will they turn? The greatest scientific libraries and centers will be gone. The art of the Louvre, the Vatican, and the Metropolitan will be ashes. In a sense Venice, which has withstood the assaults of the Adriatic Sea for a millennium, but would be vaporized in a moment, symbolizes our powerlessness before the bomb. And Jerusalem, where a few stones have stood stone upon stone since before the time of Christ, would become a bleak moonscape.

An elementary physics book would be priceless scientifically. Indeed, it might be impossible for most surviving communities in America, Europe, or the Soviet Union, to
understand anything more advanced. The human remnant in
those nations would not have to reinvent the wheel, but they
would be forced to recreate even the most elementary technology of the twentieth century. Much of the accumulated
achievements of human spirit and talent would be lost.

Perhaps it is too generous to speak of our society surviving
a nuclear war in a form that resembles a caricature of
medieval times. Nuclear war may or may not threaten the
death of the world, but it would so diminish the human condition that those who lived on would be forced back beyond
any recognizable past. The future would be theirs; but in
time, the living would envy the dead their chance, now lost
for immeasurable years, to know what it meant to be fully
human.

4

FIGHTING THE FINAL WORLD WAR

"The precariousness of command channels probably means that nuclear war would be uncontrollable, as a practical matter, shortly after the first tens of weapons are launched—regardless of what calculations political leaders might make at the time."

—John Steinbruner
Director of Foreign Policy Studies
The Brookings Institution

When the order comes, the B-52 crews rush from their barracks to their planes. In a matter of minutes, the bombers, each carrying up to 24 nuclear warheads, are airborne. The flight time to Moscow is along a prearranged path that takes at least ten hours, but it may take longer as the planes maneuver to evade Soviet air defenses. During the flight, the crew arms the bombs. A single plane can now carry more lethal power than all of the bombs dropped during World War II.

At a certain point, a coded communication orders the B-52 to proceed to its targets. Without that signal, the crew is supposed to remain in orbit over the holding point, or return to base. Once the order to proceed is given, it may not be possible to revoke it. The fabled last-minute fail-safe point of popular conception, where the plane could still be recalled, may not in fact exist.

As the B-52s enter Soviet airspace, nuclear missiles, which travel much faster, have already exploded across the Soviet Union; some of the planes will be bombing the same targets as the missiles, just to make sure. After completing their missions, and if there is enough fuel left, the pilots head for allied nations or back to the United States, looking for someplace amid the devastation where the B-52s can touch down. It seems like an endless trip, since the airmen on the plane do not know what is left of their homes and families, what kind of America they will find if they ever reach it, or whether they will have to ditch the world's most advanced bomber in an open field. All the warriors in this war could soon become its casualties.

Early in the nuclear age, analysts assumed that the prospect of just a few hydrogen bombs exploding over cities would be sufficient to deter any sane national leader from nuclear war. None of the political causes which beset this troubled world could justify an act resulting in swift retaliation that would kill tens of millions of citizens in the attacking country. Thus the concept of nuclear deterrence was born.

Despite its obvious logic, amply documented by incredible human suffering at Hiroshima and Nagasaki, and compellingly argued in many studies since then, the two superpowers have built their arsenals far beyond the simple requirements of deterrence, each fearful that the nuclear forces of the other might somehow yield significant military advantages. Some theorists argue that even perceptions of advantage might induce political capitulation from the disadvantaged side or reckless adventure from the advantaged power. Neither the American nor the Soviet military establishment has been content simply to possess the potential for devastation. Both have made assiduous preparations for actually fighting a nuclear war. Both have come to believe that their security depends upon an ability to organize massive nuclear attacks on extremely short notice—a few minutes, perhaps a few hours.

In the process of justifying large weapons inventories and elaborate peacetime preparations for using them, the two military establishments have created officially declared doctrines foreseeing the use of nuclear weapons for purposes other than deterring full-scale war. Strategic writings have imagined nuclear campaign's of extended duration conducted to serve particular political or military objectives. Though deterrence is usually set forth as the underlying purpose, the thought has nonetheless taken hold that nuclear weapons might actually be used. A decision to do so, once considered to be insane, has now been seriou'sly contemplated under certain conditions. Thousands of people stand ready to execute such a decision: submarine crews cruising beneath the oceans; young missile commanders in underground encasements; bomber crew's camped beside waiting aircraft every minute of the day. There is an inherent possibility that these arrangements for war will themselves bring it about.

The preparations for nuclear war rehearsed daily over more than two decades have created some concrete images of what it would be like. It would begin, we are told, with an unmistakable belligerent action by the opponent such as an actual launching of missile's or aircraft known to carry nuclear weapons. Electronic sensing systems would collect data from the approaching weapons and transmit it to control stations where the information would be rapidly processed to yield a diagnosis of the impending attack. Respon'sible military commanders up through the chain of command to the President himself would be alerted, and the President would be required to make the decision authorizing retaliation. A code conveying that decision and designating the form of retaliation would be sent by multiple means of communication to the immediate commanders of weapons. All this would have to occur in 20 minutes or less. Through procedures requiring the closely coordinated cooperation of individual military officers in their silos, the electronic signals would be sent to launch missiles; at a suitable point after a successful launch, their warheads would be automatically armed.

Even with attrition from mechanical failure and defen'sive enemy actions, the strategic forces available at any moment to respond to presidential instructions are more than large enough to devastate the industrial capacity and most of the principal military installations of the Soviet Union. With suitable variations in presidential instructions, the authorized attack's can, in theory, be concentrated on some particular selection of Soviet targets, and a portion of available American forces can be exempted from participating in the initial retaliation. In imagining wars of extended duration, the assumption, which may prove to be a shaky one, is that instructions

to engage in specific attacks would be issued many times to
forces that survive the initial assault. It is also assumed that
they would remain in sufficient communication contact to receive the additional instructions.

Government analysts as well as novelists have applied their
imaginations to embellish on those scenarios and have created
speculative accounts of scenes from a nuclear war. The analysts conceive of strategic situations in which the destructive
power of the American nuclear arsenal is selectively applied
to persuade belligerent Soviet leaders to abandon an aggressive adventure before a full-scale conflagration envelops
the world. The novelists invoke the enduring themes of human frailty and human heroism being played out on the edge
of massive and virtually limitless destruction. In their very
different ways, each of these strands of thought has expressed
an understandable hope that somehow nuclear weapons can
be accommodated to comprehensible human experience.

The deeper truth, however, which ultimately plagues all coherent conceptions of nuclear war, is that the destructive
power of these weapons is simply too great for human institutions to manage once that power has been unleashed. The
elaborate procedures for issuing authoritative instructions to
nuclear forces so that they can fight a purposeful military
campaign will very likely break down under the first wave of
attack. The channels of communication which link the
President and the major military commanders to the submarines, bombers, and missile silos could be substantially
destroyed; and in all likelihood, in any nuclear war, they will
be.

Americans assume, for example, that the President of the
United States has a single button he can push or a single order he can send that could set the U.S. strategic arsenal flying
to targets in the Soviet Union. Military professionals know
that the imagined button is in fact a network of interlock-
ing electronic systems and organizational arrangements. The
professionals always provide a solemn reassurance that a
President can indeed issue the necessary orders which will
result in a coordinated, even a carefully calibrated nuclear response, but Americans are seldom told that this operation,
which has never been attempted, depends on steps which cannot be fully simulated in advance. Despite all the elaborate
war-gaming, it is improbable that the strategic arsenal of either superpower would operate in accord with official designs

or decisions. Massive destruction would probably occur, but not necessarily the destruction that was intended in advance.

Military command channels will remain indefinitely vulnerable to internal confusion and external disruption. Advocates of the arms race have argued that relatively small differences in American and Soviet nuclear inventories could have major consequences for the outcome of a war and hence for the outcome of crisis bargaining. What they generally fail to say, however, is that just a few nuclear warheads, less than 1 percent of current Soviet stockpiles, could destroy the military chain of command that connects the President with his commanders and military officers, and they are the people who actually carry out the procedures to launch American nuclear weapons. Morever, 10 to 20 percent of current Soviet nuclear forces could overwhelm even the most protected chain of command presently imaginable. As John Steinbruner has written, "Fewer than 100 judiciously targeted nuclear weapons could so severely damage U.S. communications facilities and command centers that form the military chain of command that the actions of individual weapons commanders could no longer be controlled or coordinated. Some bomber crews, submarine officers, and ICBM silo launcher officers could undertake very damaging retaliation"—but only on their own. Steinbruner, who calls this phenomenon "nuclear decapitation," concludes that as few as 50 Soviet nuclear weapons could make it impossible for anyone "to direct U.S. strategic forces to coherent purposes."

As few as one to five Soviet warheads exploded at high altitude would blanket the United States with electromagnetic pulses of enormous power. These pulses could damage or destroy the solid state circuitry at the heart of most American military technology and communications. In this context, the details of precise nuclear balance in every area of weaponry may prove to be relatively insignificant. The utility of individual weapons is questionable in a post-attack period, since there may be no surviving military organization capable of controlling them.

Shortly after the onset of a nuclear war, with central authorities incapable of functioning, surviving weapons commanders would be left to their own judgments. The crews of submarines, bombers, and missile silos, who would be isolated, confused, frightened, and provoked, would have to decide for themselves what they would do. Some of them probably would improvise and execute attacks as they assume higher authorities may have wished. The possibility of sustained purpose would die in the initial assault.

Much of the information about the authority to launch submarine missiles, for example, is classified. But it can be assumed that a launch depends on a multiple lock system under which several officers would have to act in concert after an order from the command structure in the United States. It can also be assumed, however, that at some point after the communication link with the United States is broken, a submarine crew could fire the missiles without specific authorization from the President or his successor. What would happen during a crisis if the crew of a submarine was attacked unsuccessfully, and at the same time, was receiving no message on standard communication channels? What if that lonely crew had reason to believe that war had broken out, even though they had not been officially told? What if the communications silence continued over many hours or many days? No one can be sure of the answer, but some submarine under these circumstances could initiate nuclear war on its own. And a single submarine alone is capable of mounting a war larger than any conflict in human history. Finally, if a communications link is broken in the first hours after a war starts, a submarine commander might not know if American and Soviet leaders had agreed to a truce. Fearful that the war was still raging, a commander could decide that he had waited long enough, launch his missiles at Soviet targets, and shatter the truce. Both sides understand this possibility and both sides have to doubt that any truce could be effectively enforced. Any nuclear war is likely to escalate to all-out nuclear war.

In short, there is a major distinction between the procedures for handling nuclear weapons in peacetime and the procedures for handling them in crisis and in war. In peacetime, the principal challenge is to prevent any accidental or unauthorized use of the weapons by military officials who have immediate control over them, and to prevent them from falling into the hands of terrorists. Safeguards are in place to ensure that individuals cannot misuse their access to the launch of a thermonuclear warhead which could kill millions of people. These safeguards dominate peacetime military operations, even the ones designed to train people for war. The controls are as absolute as it is humanly possible to make them, but in all likelihood they are too cumbersome to be preserved under conditions of a nuclear battle. For the forces in that battle, the refined calculus of careful control would become a distant discredited doctrine, an ivory tower theory far removed from the conning tower reality of their submarines. The men in missile silos and in bombers would be driven by immediate operational problems. Their judgments would be dominated by despair; they would be at once the most powerful and the most powerless soldiers in history.

There are many other ways the system could collapse and bring on conflict or escalation. How would the United States react if its intelligence sensors suddenly went blind in the midst of a serious confrontation? What should surviving decision makers do if, during such a confrontation, the President and his principal advisers are killed in an accident that is conventional in character but mysterious in origin? What is the appropriate reaction if spy satellites in space are systematically shot down in an attack that is limited to outer space? There are hundreds of questions like these that have no clear answers because the nuclear age has no precedent in our experience of warfare.

Such questions confound limited war theorists, who argue that we may face threats of limited nuclear engagements and that resisting such threats requires well-developed capabilities to respond in kind. On this basis, they justify increases in the number of weapons and expensive efforts to modernize them. But the single, overwhelming defect in the conception of limited nuclear conflict is the vulnerability of the men and machines supposed to direct the battle. Although individual weapons can be protected against nuclear attack, the chain of command cannot be preserved. The vulnerability of both sides to preemptive strikes against command organizations is too great to allow either side any serious attempt at limited nuclear operations.

These stark facts represent a fatal contradiction in the evolution of strategic policy. They turn notions of fighting a calibrated nuclear war into nothing more than overintellectualized myths. The arguments so prominent in current policy for preparing to fight enduring, precisely defined military campaigns with nuclear weapons fall before a simple military reality: Since the destruction of the opposing command system is the single most effective thing that can be done to reduce the opponent's strategic power, it is almost certain to be the *first thing* that would be done by any country provoked enough to use nuclear weapons in the first place. Should one side or the other be foolish enough to initiate an attack and still leave the opponent's command system sufficiently undamaged to organize a deliberately planned retaliation, then the retaliatory strike would likely be aimed at those directly responsible for the initial attack. Therefore, we must expect that both sides' strategic command organizations would be destroyed in the initial exchanges of a nuclear war, and that surviving forces could not be deployed with a fine sense of graduated response. Knowing this, responsible military commanders would feel pressed to commit themselves to full-scale retaliation at the very outset of a serious nuclear attack. The idea of limited nuclear war, used as a rationale for large inventories of weapons, is not a feasible or a responsible policy once war has become a serious prospect.

This simple fact has recently been recognized and the problem of command, C^{3}I control, communication, and intelligence—"C^{3}I" in Pentagon jargon—has been defined as the top priority for the United States strategic program. At the moment, however, the implications of that priority are completely unclear, and quite literally our military planners do not yet know what to do about it.

Despite all the talk about the role of nuclear weapons bolstering national resolve under the challenge of a crisis, and despite an unfortunate habit of using the alerts of nuclear forces to send diplomatic signals of such resolve, the stark truth is that the United States is not technically prepared, and probably cannot become prepared, to realistically wage the theoretical scenario of limited nuclear conflict. Neither, in all probability, is the Soviet Union. Government policy declarations to the contrary do not change that truth; they only state aspirations to change it. They are wishes, as it were, that have not yet been accomplished and almost certainly cannot be, however keenly nuclear strategists may pine for them. The strategists may imagine a coherent nuclear conflict; but in the real world, the manipulation of nuclear forces in the heat of crisis is a provocative and irresponsible way of communicating national resolve. Given the vulnerabilities of both sides to initial attack, any serious alert during a major crisis may signal an impending attack and trigger an uncontrollable process that escalates into all-out nuclear war, no matter what political leaders may think they are doing.

Mercifully, we have been spared any test of the behavior of fully developed and fully deployed nuclear forces under such circumstances. The only major confrontation of the nuclear era, the Cuban missile crisis of 1962, came before current sophisticated arsenals were in place. Before we stumble into a mutual test of nuclear gamesmanship and fail at it, we must recognize that nuclear weapons can play only a very restricted role in our national security. They deter a nuclear attack by means of a countervailing nuclear threat. They can do little more than that, and it is courting disaster to imagine that they can.

To count on the possibility of limited nuclear war is to gamble civilization on an untried and unworkable set of hypotheses. The uncertainty which shrouds the details of fighting a nuclear war does not prevent an overall judgment about whether it is truly thinkable. No nation and no military organization can fight such a war and survive as a coherent entity. Although we have never observed the death of an entire society, we know historically that it has happened in the past. The United States, the Soviet Union, and the allies on both sides could not sustain the sudden massive destruction of full-scale nuclear war and still exist as functioning societies.

Yet the preparations for nuclear war-fighting at so-called thinkable levels have been accelerated by the current administration. In the first five days of March, 1982 President Reagan and the entire U.S. military establishment participated in an exercise, code-named "Ivy League," under which they played out a measured, and initially limited nuclear war. It was the first such comprehensive nuclear war game by the United States since 1956. During the mock exchange, hundreds of Soviet missiles struck the United States. The war had escalated from an initial Soviet strike with tactical nuclear weapons against a U.S. ship in the North Atlantic; on the fourth day of the crisis the Soviets launched a full-scale missile attack against American military targets. The President died in the White House situation room during the Soviet assault on the communication and command structure. Power shifted to the Vice-President, who was airborne in the specially equipped Boeing 747 known as the "Doomsday Plane." It shifted again, and then once more, to Cabinet officials at secret bases in Massachusetts and Texas. In the event of a genuine attack, however, the President or Vice-President in the Doomsday Plane might very well be knocked out of the sky by a nuclear airburst or forced down when there were no tankers left to refuel the plane. Like the returning B-52s, it is not clear where or whether it would land. All the participants in a nuclear war, including the generals and the Commander-in-Chief, are likely to become victims as well.

Yet in the face of the catastrophic consequences apparent to both American and Soviet leaders, preparations like these for fighting with nuclear weapons are going forward in both Washington and Moscow. The irony is that this elaborate, expensive mutual anticipation of nuclear conflict could ultimately produce it. In short, the Soviet-American nuclear arsenals, and their command systems, are a technological nightmare.

A mutual freeze on Soviet and American arsenals followed by reductions in nuclear weapons will not automatically solve these underlying problems in the United States strategic weapons posture, but such measures are essential first steps. A freeze can reverse the process of anticipating war that now besets the two superpowers. By itself, it can send a clear signal that at last we are on the road to peace. The reductions negotiated during a freeze can eliminate the most provocative and vulnerable weapons, the lethal toys of the first-strike theorists who imagine conditions for nuclear war, and who by their imaginings contribute to the atmosphere that may bring it about. But in the absence of a freeze, even negotiations for reductions still permit each side to build more and more weapons while both sides talk and talk. This course totally fails to deal with the continuing climate of war anticipation. A freeze can anticipate peace and thereby do more than any other policy to secure America and the world from the overhanging threat of the nuclear storm.

5

THE ILLUSION OF CIVIL DEFENSE

"Deep shelters would become deep tombs."
—Admiral Noel Gayler
Former Director,
National Security Agency

On March 29, 1982, the Reagan administration announced that it would ask Congress to approve a new $4.2 billion program for civil defense against nuclear attack. The program calls for relocating the entire urban population away from targeted cities and into the countryside, where they would be crammed into basements and improvised fallout shelters. Plans to build deep shelters to protect industrial workers from the effects of a nuclear blast are under consideration. This program is part of a nuclear war-fighting strategy which assumes that such conflict is not only possible, but potentially winnable. Even its proponents admit that a civil defense undertaking on this scale is without precedent in this country; there is very little proof that it would actually work in practice. As James Holton, the administration's civil defense spokesman, concedes, "This is a complicated business."

Civil defense programs are also a dubious and dangerous business, which have been tried and judged a failure many times in the past. The new proposal is the latest chapter in a long and beleaguered history of discarded programs that supposedly would save lives in a nuclear holocaust. The experience of this history reinforces the logic of common sense that any such hope is essentially illusory. Only episodically in the past four decades has civil defense been taken seriously.

In the 1950s there were plans to evacuate cities in the event of warnings of a Soviet bomber attack. The bombers would have taken ten hours to fly from the Soviet Union to their targets, and five hours of warning to the public seemed likely. Highways were marked as evacuation routes. Although it was clear even then that far more than the allotted five hours would be needed to move any substantial number of people out of any major city, the plan soon became obsolete due to the advances of weapons technology. By the time the plan was in place, missiles with a 30-minute flight time were replacing the bombers that gave hours of warning.

By the early 1960s, defense planners recognized that the only possible protection for people close to likely targets would come from "blast shelters," which would be prohibitively expensive. And even at a cost of hundreds of dollars per person per shelter, they still offered no assurance that the occupants would not be cooked and then entombed inside under tons of debris deposited on top of the shelter.

In the absence of other alternatives, civil defense next focused on fallout shelters in suburbs and in rural areas, where layers of dirt or underground basements could shield survivors of the blast from the radioactivity that would otherwise poison them. During the Berlin crisis in 1961, leaflets were available from post offices about fallout shelters, and many shelters were stocked with water and biscuits. Suddenly Americans were debating who would have a fallout shelter and who would not and how they would be protected from others looking for refuge. Some families bought guns to keep neighbors out of their backyard bunkers; they seemed to believe that a man's shelter was his castle. The Kennedy administration, which briefly emphasized the shelter program, soon decided to let it wither away because of its impracticality. The water and the biscuits stored in the tin drums in the underground hallways spoiled unnoticed as the years passed.

Inside and outside the government, civil defense came to be viewed as inherently unworkable and even unethical. No combination of shelters and evacuation plans could reduce to any acceptable level the human casualties from thousands of nuclear explosions many times more powerful than the Hiroshima bomb. Military planners in both Republican and Democratic administrations emphasized the need to prevent nuclear war, not to prepare citizens for the day when it would come. But as the 1980s began, a number of analysts and officials, ignoring the lessons of recent history, started to look upon nuclear conflict as something that could be handled with adequate planning. The resurgence of civil defense reflects the view that nuclear war can be fought and won and that unless we develop elaborate means for protecting our citizens, a U.S. nuclear war-fighting strategy will not be credible. The Federal Emergency Management Agency, which is responsible for the new civil defense program, has issued the reassuring consolation that "the United States could survive nuclear attack and go on to recover within a relatively few years."

Today, supporters of civil defense face an even more impossible task than when they failed in the past. Soviet weapons now include not just a few new ICBMs and older bombers, as was the case in the early 1960s, but 7500 warheads, many of one megaton or more. They possess almost more warheads than we have cities and towns. And each one-megaton warhead is 67 times as large in explosive power as the Hiroshima bomb; even cities with millions of inhabitants could be overkilled by such warheads. There is no conceivable way of defending people against an all-out Soviet nuclear attack by relying on shelters within city limits. As a consequence, strategic planners favoring civil defense have returned to the old idea of evacuation, and not just of cities, but of smaller towns as well. And since there will be no more than a 30-minute warning of the actual attack, they assume that it will come only after a preliminary crisis that lasts several days and that signals the likelihood of nuclear war.

On the basis of that scenario, the administration plans to develop a Crisis Relocation Plan which, it contends, could significantly improve the odds of survival for Americans in a nuclear war. The plan involves the temporary relocation of people from "high-risk" areas to safer areas during periods of international crisis. High-risk areas are defined as metropolitan areas of 50,000 or more population as well as areas near military installations. The safer places would become "host areas" during an emergency and would provide care and fallout protection for urban refugees. In short, all Americans would be divided into "hosts" and "evacuees"; survival would

depend on an orderly flow of highway traffic at a time of incredible tension, chaos, and near madness.

In fact, the crisis relocation program is not really primarily
directed to save lives. The administration is using it as a tool
in the contest for strategic advantage with the Soviet Union.
In a sense, it is only an attempt to match what the Russians
are doing. American advocates now justify civil defense by
pointing to what they regard as an advancing Soviet program.
The administration asserts that the much larger Soviet investment in civil defense of $2 billion a year over the past decade
indicates that the Soviets are preparing not only to survive,
but to prevail in a nuclear war. Yet according to a 1978 Central Intelligence Agency report, $2 billion is not what the So-
viets actually spend, but an estimate of what they would
spend if they paid their workers at the same wage scale as the
United States. It goes without saying that Soviet wages are
not equal to American wages. Moreover, the administration is
planning to spend much more than a few hundred million
dollars a year for its new program. Several billion dollars will
be close to the cost in the foreseeable future, perhaps more in
real terms than the Soviets themselves devote to protecting
their own civilians.

Civil defense advocates respond that the Soviet program,
even in its less imposing reality, could permit Soviet leaders
to resort to a first strike during a crisis, while keeping the fatalities due to American retaliation at an "acceptably low
level." Richard Pipes, the senior Soviet expert in the National
Security Council, has defined the meaning of that level. He
suggests that the Soviets might be willing to sacrifice 20 million people, the same number they lost in World War II, in
order to wage a nuclear war. In effect, the argument is that
the Soviets would not mind if the worst six years in their history repeated themself in approximately six minutes. And
even the estimate of "only" 20 million Soviet dead rests on
the remote possibility that Soviet civil defense would work all
but perfectly.

Even many of its supporters recognize that American evacuation planning is not, in any meaningful sense, a workable
part of the nuclear war game, but merely an attempt to
manifest our determination to match a tactic in the paper
plans of the Soviet Union. The 1978 CIA study discounts the
notion that the Soviets believe that their civil defense system
gives them a strategic edge: "They cannot have confidence

. . . in the degree of protection their civil defenses would afford them, given the many uncertainties attendant to a nuclear exchange. We do not believe that the Soviets' present civil defenses would embolden them deliberately to expose the U.S.S.R. to a higher risk of nuclear attack." Must we strive to duplicate every capability which the Soviets claim, even when their plans can't work and we know only too well that ours can't work either?

Nevertheless, the administration persists in the view that in a heavy nuclear attack on military, urban, and industrial targets in the mid-1980s, evacuation could save tens of millions of Americans. The Federal Emergency Management Agency asserts: "Performance in a large-scale mid-1980s attack would be on the order of 80% survival of the U.S. population, if the bulk of risk area population had been evacuated to host areas prior to attack, and if fallout protection had been developed and other crisis action taken." The data and assumptions on which this estimate is based are alternately unclear and unreliable. What is clear is that the estimate rests on a series of highly improbable conditions: a range of "ifs" unlikely ever to occur in the real world. Upon examination, evacuation planning becomes a theater of the absurd, in which everything we intuitively understand about human behavior is turned on its head.

The first assumption behind the rosy estimate of 80 percent survival is, in the administration's words, that "it is *likely* we would have a week's warning time because the Soviets must protect the bulk of their urban population by evacuation, and the intelligence community estimates that it would take a week or more to evacuate Soviet cities and develop fallout protection for evacuees in surrounding rural areas." But most of our own military planners would regard it as unwise to discount any possibility of a surprise Soviet attack, or to rely on the hope that the Soviets would conveniently give us ample warning. Even the administration knows that its relocation plan would fail in all but an openly planned assault visible seven days in advance. But even assuming the "right" kind of attack seemed to be in the offing, a mass evacuation of target sites could well provoke precisely the nuclear war from which it purports to protect us. Can you imagine how strategic planners in Moscow would react if their spy satellites saw streams of cars crawling along clogged highways, fleeing from New York City toward the Adirondacks? Rather than improving this country's nuclear war preparedness, crisis relocation could intensify Soviet fears of an American first strike. Rather than providing stability in a crisis, which is the ultimate aim of deterrence, evacuation will reinforce the temptation to yield a "hair-trigger" mentality. The plans for crisis relocation defy imagination and deny the logic of strategic deterrence, according to which neither side should have any incentive to strike first in a crisis, and neither side should behave so provocatively that it induces the very attack if hopes to deter.

But even with adequate warning, and even if civil defense did not prove counterproductive, evacuation would require the highest degree of cooperation and order at exactly the time when virtually all Americans would feel themselves threatened with instant extinction. Even the heroic would be tempted to lose hope, at the very least. In the words of Robert Lifton: "The ultimate threat posed by nuclear weapons is not only death but meaninglessness: an unknown death by an unimaginable weapon." No one can predict how people would react. The federal civil defense agency optimistically expects public cooperation because the "experience in both peacetime and wartime evacuation is that most people will comply with official instructions, provided that these are understandable and make sense in terms of improving chances for human survival." But there is no experience with the kind of national disaster that nuclear war would represent. The capacity to evacuate a few thousand people from a flooded area hardly suggests that a hundred million or more could be readily moved out of every major city and most medium-size towns.

The new civil defense proposal is not an effective plan, but a facade. It relies on so many questionable predictions that it raises serious questions about the common sense of civil defense planners. It assumes that American citizens would be willing to leave their homes, to risk total separation from family, friends, and neighbors, all in order to prove to the Soviets that we were serious about fighting a war or to make a marginal improvement in our bargaining position in a crisis. The effort to implement crisis relocation could easily have exactly the opposite effect. Millions of Americans would react by urging our government not to risk a war because it could only mean national suicide. Millions more might understandably panic. The net effect would be to persuade the Soviets that this country was weak, divided, disorganized, and frightened. Facing this prospect, no rational American President would ever order a mass evacuation; even as the threat of war intensified, Washington would issue soothing words about our capacity to deter an attack. Whether or not war was averted, the expensive civil defense planning would prove to be a waste. Even if an evacuation were ordered, the least likely possiblity is that it would go according to plan. Many citizens will not be able to leave their homes, especially if they are poor, sick, elderly, or pregnant; others will simply reject the idea of evacuation. It is by no means certain that even those who do leave would cooperate with each other during the relocation effort. Anyone who has sat in rush-hour traffic while commuting from a city to the suburbs understands that crisis relocation could quickly descend into mass hysteria. The civil defense agency's advice to people trapped in such situations is cheerily nonresponsive: "If you get caught in a traffic jam, turn off your engine, remain in your car, listen for official instructions, and be patient. Do not get out of line to find an alternate route. All routes will be crowded."

A California State Senator who heard a federal official enthusiastically describe a program to move 19 million Californians into the desert asked one blunt question: "Have you gone insane?" If the insanity ever actually went into effect, and if the evacuation went well, the leadership of the Soviet Union could undo it simply by threatening and finally by destroying the evacuated population, as well as its water, energy, and food supplies, which the Soviets certainly have the weapons to do. With all these perils it is incredibly foolish to believe that any crisis relocation plan can work. Physicians for Social Responsiblity states categorically: "There is no effective civil defense. The blast, thermal, and radiation effects would kill even those in shelters, and the fallout would reach those who had been evacuated." The relocation plan presumes that there would be safe "host areas"; but in grim truth, the entire nation would be at risk from thousands of warheads that could blast, burn, or contaminate all of America.

The civil defense agency thinks the risk can be countered by building antiradiation fallout shelters in the countryside. Indeed, a Deputy Under Secretary of Defense, T. K. Jones, concludes that the United States could fully recover from an all-out nuclear war with the Soviet Union in "two to four years"; as he states, "Everybody's going to make it if there are enough shovels to go around. . . . Dig a hole, cover it up with a few doors and then throw three feet of dirt on top. It's the dirt that does it." But would there be enough shovels to do it, enough doors to go around, and ground soft enough for digging in northern states, if an attack came in the midst of winter? And what about the food, water, medicine, radios, insulation, heat, waterproofing, and sewage removal for the people inside the shelters? As Senator Paul Tsongas put it at a hearing of the Senate Arms Control Subcommittee in Washington, D.C., "I think we should get the T. K. Joneses of this Administration out before the TV cameras, before the media and let the people of this country take a good hard look. . . . What is interesting about the discussion that takes place in this city on these issues is that it is remarkably amoral. In fact it is fashionable in the arms control community not to allow emotions or feelings to intervene in one's analytical process and there is a premium put on having an amoral capacity—not immoral, just simply devoid of moral responsibility. That attitude, I would argue . . . is limited to this city. If you go out around this country and you talk about these issues, people will think you are crazy . . . If the Administration wants to engage in right-wing ideology and destroy the economy, I suppose we can live with it. But if they wish to engage in right-wing ideology and destroy my children, I for one am not going to stand by."

Dr. Irwin Redlener, who has studied crisis relocation for Physicians for Social Responsibility, says that civil defense planners ignore essential differences between people fleeing a city in the face of a hurricane and fleeing a city about to be obliterated by a nuclear bomb. Crisis relocation "requires the evacuated families to shovel piles of dirt around the buildings to which they are assigned in order to make them radiation-safe, but does not speak to how this might be accomplished during the winter months in a northern climate. Even in the national model areas [such as Plattsburgh, New York] where it has been rather fully developed, there is no real provision for the management of hospitalized patients in the target sites or for the redirection of essential services such as food."

In addition there is no way to predict how different areas of the country would be affected by radiation. That would depend on unpredictable variables: whether the bombs were detonated on the ground or in the air; the size and type of bombs used; the condition of the weather; and the direction of the wind. On the assumption that half the warheads would be groundbursts, which deliver greater radiation than airbursts, the U.S. Arms Control and Disarmament Agency (ACDA) calculated in 1979, as shown in Figure 1, that the short-term radiation fallout from an all-out nuclear attack would expose 80 percent of the urban population and 75 percent of the rural population to radiation doses of 100 rem or more—levels at which death or serious illness will result.

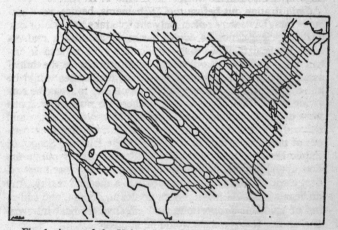

Fig. 1. Areas of the United States exposing persons in the open to radiation of 100 rem or more after an all-out nuclear attack

For many of those who survive the blast and fire effects, there will be no safe or scientific way to gauge how long to stay in their shelters, at least in the initial period after the blast. If radio or other communications come to be restored, guidance might become available, but it would hardly be music to anyone's ears. According to the ACDA study, even those in the most radiation-proof fallout shelters will face lengthy stays of "sheltered" life; and to avoid a dangerous threshold of radiation exposure, they would have to spend as much as 100 percent of the first month in shelters. In the second month, they could spend perhaps 75 percent of their time in the shelters and the rest of the time somewhere else indoors. In the third month, they could leave the shelter, but they might still have to spend 75 percent of their time indoors and only 25 percent outdoors. Incredibly, a 1980 study sponsored by the Department of Energy suggested that the long-term effects of cancer and other radiation disease were not that bad; after all, they could be mitigated by choosing only older people to go outside in search of food and water during the exposure period, while younger persons stayed inside the shelter. The elderly, the study said in effect, would naturally die sooner anyway.

Civil defense predictions of high survival rates have another fatal flaw: they reflect only the inherent promise of our medical science, not its actual performance after a real attack. Medical facilities and supplies are concentrated in urban areas and nearly all would be wiped out in the initial assault. The vast majority of physicians and nurses would be killed or injured and would hardly be on call to treat the surviving population. Even in areas where no nuclear weapons were exploded, radioactive fallout would prevent doctors and nurses from reaching the injured and the dying for long periods of time. According to the Dean of the Harvard School of Public Health, Dr. Howard Hiatt, "Recent talk by public figures about winning or even surviving a nuclear war must reflect a widespread failure to appreciate a medical reality. Any nuclear war would inevitably cause death, disease, and suffering of epidemic proportions, and effective medical intervention on any realistic scale would be impossible."

It is important to heed such physicians, not only for their medical expertise, but also for their experience in emergency treatment. Doctors who have examined the problem agree that there is no possible plan that can practically counter the effects of radiation. According to Patricia Lindop, Professor of Radiation Biology at the Medical College of London, and Joseph Rotblat, former President of the British Institute of Radiology, "The ubiquitous nature of radioactive fallout, the unpredictability of its distribution, and its persistence render useless any medical planning for dealing with the casualties of a nuclear attack. Underestimating the radiation problem for man himself, let alone for the food and resources on which his long-term survival depends, makes civil defense planning for the post-nuclear attack period a travesty of morality."

In disregard of the scientific and medical evidence, civil defense planners profess public faith in a concept that is implausible at best and irresponsible at worst. The new civil defense theology is at the heart of the difference between those who believe a nuclear war is fightable and winnable and those who believe it would mean Soviet-American suicide. Treating relocation as a realistic option for defense against nuclear war is little more than a subliminal means to condition Americans to prepare for and accept the unthinkable. Nuclear war fighting can never be a rational instrument of national policy.

Supporters of the nuclear weapons freeze understand the futility of civil defense and the mentality behind it. They have been active in holding hearings on civil defense planning in their own communities. A hearing in Cambridge, Massachusetts, left City Council members with a sense of disbelief and horror. The Council concluded: "[T]he sole means of protecting Cambridge citizens from nuclear warfare would be for nations with nuclear arms to destroy those arms and renounce their use." The Council then told its local emergency management director not to participate in further civil defense planning. In Boulder, Colorado, a citizens' committee determined that the crisis relocation plan was "unworkable, misleading, and a gross misdirection of resources." They rejected the plan because it offered the public a false sense of security and emphasized that federal efforts should be directed towards arms control rather than civil defense.

Such hearings can, and should, be held in each of the hundreds of cities considered to be prime targets in a nuclear war. The hearings can educate the public about the reality of a nuclear war, the unreality of civil defense, and the necessity of a nuclear weapons freeze. And once a freeze is in place, there will be a new and different climate, in which far-fetched wargames will be seen for the menacing fantasies they really are.

6

THE NEXT ROUND IN
THE ARMS RACE

> "We have gone on piling weapon upon
> weapon, missile upon missile, new levels of
> destructiveness upon old ones, helplessly, al-
> most involuntarily, like victims of some sort
> of hypnotism, like men in a dream, like lem-
> mings headed for the sea."
>
> —George F. Kennan, former U.S.
> Ambassador to Moscow

In 1946, the United States offered to consign all nuclear weapons to the control of an international organization. The plan, named for its author, Bernard Baruch, was immediately rejected by Soviet leaders. They could not be expected, they said, to rely on an international agency dominated by the United States. They were unwilling to drop out of the nuclear weapons race after America had already run it and won it, and they had just barely begun.

For nearly a decade, there were no meaningful arms control negotiations between the United States and Stalin's Russia. With the onset of the Eisenhower administration, Soviet leaders interpreted the massive retaliation doctrine announced by Secretary of State John Foster Dulles as pointing toward an American capability to strike first with nuclear weapons, even in a conventional conflict. Within a few years, American leaders were worrying about a missile gap that would leave the United States vulnerable to Soviet attack. Each side engaged in nuclear brinksmanship, and both sides were wrong about the other's capabilities. For example, the United States was never behind in strategic missiles and soon was far ahead. At the United Nations Disarmament Commission, negotiators for each superpower regularly presented plans for general and complete disarmament which the other superpower interpreted as self-serving.

Throughout this period, and well into the 1960s, the United States had unquestionable superiority in nuclear weapons. But despite an early monopoly and a continuing clear advantage, the U.S. never took up the temptation to finish off the Soviets before they could retaliate in kind. Although Presidents made the threat, as in Iran in 1946, and during the Korean War truce talks in 1953—and we faced the threat of nuclear war during the Cuban missile crisis—the United States never seriously contemplated eradicating communism with a single nuclear blow. Perhaps few other countries in history would have been as restrained. Who believes that if the tables had been turned, the Soviets would have shown similar forbearance? Still, American restraint had its limits. In those days no administration was willing to concede nuclear parity to the Soviet Union. We were far ahead, and it was assumed that we should be, and that we always would be. Every American disarmament proposal was founded on that assumption—and foundered on it.

At the Geneva Summit Conference in 1955, President Eisenhower proposed an "Open Skies" program, under which the Soviets and the Americans would exchange blueprints of all military forces and bases and permit overflights to verify the data. The Soviets rejected this American initiative as well. They responded that the proposal, which had been hurriedly conceived at the personal insistence of the President, might decrease rather than increase international security because it would enable the United States to ferrett out the soft spots of the Soviet deterrent. Such information, which the Soviets could also have obtained about American defenses, could have encouraged any adversary to plan a first strike. The specter of John Foster Dulles's doctrine of massive retaliation haunted the discussions; but it is far from certain that, upon reflection, the Eisenhower administration would have agreed to its own proposal.

The only real advance in arms control in the 1950s was in

the area of nuclear testing. Prolonged negotiations worked out some of the details of verification which later became the basis for the 1963 Test Ban Treaty. That treaty, negotiated for the United States by W. Averell Harriman and signed by President Kennedy, banned all nuclear tests in the atmosphere, in space, or underwater. In the same period, the Kennedy administration also achieved a "hot-line" agreement, to ensure that Soviet and American leaders could communiqué in the event of a crisis.

In the fall of 1963 President Kennedy directed his arms control negotiators to prepare a proposal for a Soviet-American freeze on the "number and character of strategic and defensive vehicles." Upon taking office, Lyndon Johnson approved that offer, which was put forward in January 1964. The Soviets rejected it almost immediately, because they calculated that it would freeze their forces into a position of permanent inferiority. At that time, the United States had over 7000 strategic nuclear warheads, 1100 strategic missiles, and over 1000 strategic bombers. The Soviets had less than one-fifth as many.

The next round of arms talks opened under the cloud of a new strategic threat: the impending deployment of antiballistic missiles, which in theory could threaten the policy of mutually assured destruction called MAD, which held that the key to deterring nuclear war was the ability of the other side to retaliate overwhelmingly. If the ABM could protect both missile bases and cities, that doctrine would collapse. The Johnson administration called for negotiations on ABM and other issues, including strategic arms limitation. Thus the SALT talks were born, but the Soviet invasion of Czechoslovakia in August 1968 led to their immediate cancellation.

By 1970 a new administration had resumed the discussions; President Nixon claimed that his purpose was a sufficiency, not a superiority, of nuclear forces. Nonetheless, the administration refused to pursue the idea of a comprehensive freeze on offensive and defensive strategic systems, which the Senate had overwhelmingly approved by a vote of 73 to 6. Instead, the President and his National Security Advisor Henry Kissinger held talks in Moscow in 1972, where they concluded the SALT I and ABM treaties. The ABM treaty limited each country to a maximum of two ABM sites. The United States has built one site, but has never chosen to make it operational, since the capability of the ABM proved to be more theoretical than real.

The second round of SALT nearly culminated at the Vladivostok conference in 1974. The new President, Gerald Ford, agreed in principle to a SALT II treaty. Final negotiations, however, were postponed when the President faced a challenge for renomination from former California Governor Ronald Reagan, who was skeptical of any agreement with the Russians. When the Carter administration took office the delay continued while the administration asked the Soviets for deep reductions in nuclear arsenals. The Soviets interpreted the specific cuts in the Carter proposal as clearly tilted in America's favor and dismissed it out of hand. After two years the Carter administration finally negotiated a treaty only slightly better than the Vladivostok agreement. The treaty was hardly restrictive for the United States. Although it set a ceiling on many weapons, that ceiling would have no effect on planned U.S. strategic programs. But even this treaty proved politically weak because, as the 1980 election neared, Ronald Reagan's skepticism about agreements with the Soviets largely took hold of the Republican Party and aroused ready sympathy with many Democrats as well.

One criticism of SALT was that the Soviets could not be trusted to keep their word. Opponents of arms control charged there had been serious violations of SALT I. But most experts found little in the record to justify that accusation; in truth, there had been minor violations on both sides. As the States Department said in a 1979 report on alleged Soviet breaches of the SALT agreements: "In each case the United States has raised, the activity in question has either ceased or additional information has allayed our concern." The Russians have held to the ABM treaty, and today they are not taking actions that would undercut the terms of SALT II, even though it has never been ratified by the Senate. There is little dispute about American, and for that matter Soviet, ability to verify arms control agreements, although technological advances could erode that ability if the arms race proceeds unchecked in the years ahead. Wisconsin Congressman Les Aspin, a respected authority on defense and arms control, has concluded that, at least under current circumstances, the odds against successful Soviet cheating on arms control limits are "extremely high."

Simultaneously with the Salt II negotiations, the United

States, the Soviet Union and Great Britain were engaged in negotiations for a Comprehensive Test Ban Treaty (CTB) to prevent underground nuclear tests in addition to the air, space and underwater tests already prohibited by the Test Ban Treaty of 1963. Such a treaty would represent a freeze on nuclear testing and would be an important step toward ending the nuclear arms race. During the negotiations the Soviets agreed in principle to install unmanned monitoring stations and even to permit manned inspection procedures on their territory—a major breakthrough in the traditional Soviet resistance to on-site inspection and an important advance in our ability to verify arms control agreements. The CTB treaty is still within reach, although the Reagan Administration suspended the negotiations. The excuse used for the suspension was that the Administration was unwilling to procede with such negotiations while the Soviet Union was engaged in misconduct in other areas. As ACDA Director Eugene Rostow stated, "International conditions have not been propitious and are not now propitious for immediate action on this worthy project." Meanwhile, underground nuclear testing continues to feed the nuclear arms race.

Over the past generation, in piecemeal fashion, weapon by weapon, the superpowers have sought to negotiate limits and rules for the arms race. We have never had a comprehensive freeze proposal at a point of approximate nuclear parity between the two sides. We are at that point now, but there has been no progress on arms control under the Reagan administration. Tragically, the collapse of the process comes at the very moment when the world is poised at the starting line of a new round in the arms race, one that resurrects the specter of a first strike and that could shake the nuclear balance in unpredictable and uncontrollable ways. Lemming-like, the superpowers now approach a decisive juncture in history, which may be the final opportunity to impose meaningful restraints on the nuclear arsenals of both sides. Yet today each side rejects the arms control posture of the other, while all of us become dramatically less secure as we near the point of no return in nuclear escalation.

In late March 1982, in response to the Kennedy-Hatfield freeze resolution, President Reagan said in effect that we have to build more nuclear bombs in order to reduce the number of nuclear bombs. One of us immediately labeled that approach for what it is—"voodoo arms control"—meaning that you must have more in order to have less. The administration claims we are behind the Soviets, but no one in authority, including President Reagan, would trade our deterrent for the Soviet forces. This nation is fully capable of defending itself. And if the administration thinks we can now build more while the Soviets will do nothing, then it is dangerously naive about the Russians.

Indeed, the sputtering pace of arms control is paralleled by the accelerating tempo of the arms race. In nuclear weapons lore, Newton's third law of motion has proved to be the first law of upward movement in the arms race: for every action, there is an equal and opposite reaction. The course in American-Soviet nuclear weapons history can be taught the ten easy steps of the following time chart showing the first date of testing for warheads and the first date of deployment for missiles and other delivery vehicles:

United States	Weapon	Soviet Union
1945	Atomic Bomb	1949
1948	Intercontinental Bomber	1955
1952	Hydrogen Bomb	1955
1958	Intercontinental Ballistic Missile (ICBM)	1957
1958	Satellite in Orbit	1957
1960	Submarine-Launched Ballistic Missile (SLBM)	1968
1964	Multiple Warhead Missile	1973
1972	Anti-Ballistic Missile (ABM)	1968
1970	Multiple Independently Targetable Re-entry Vehicle (MIRV)	1975
1982	Long Range Cruise Missile	198__

Instead of learning from this history, the Reagan administration seems bent on condemning America to repeat it. At this writing, it has postponed the start of strategic arms control negotiations for 15 months, which is, ironically, the number of minutes a President might have to decide to retaliate against an apparent Soviet attack. We have been told that before we talk and agree, we must close a window of vulnerability. The vulnerability idea rests on the thesis that the Soviet Union has made such significant advances in weapons capability that a small portion of its strategic forces could knock out all American land-based missiles, leaving the United States in a position where we would either have to surrender or launch a retaliatory strike against Soviet population centers and risk the same level of retaliation in return. This first-strike scenario envisions thousands of Soviet warheads fired against our 1052 land-based intercontinental missile systems in fixed silos.

The success of a Soviet first strike, even against this fraction of our overall strategic forces, is so implausible that for the Soviets to attempt it would amount, in former Defense Secretary Harold Brown's words, to "a cosmic roll of the dice." The Soviet leadership would have to be confident of a series of far-fetched assumptions before venturing a first strike. Soviet leaders would have to believe that they could carry out a nearly perfect attack. This would entail split-second timing and the coordinated launch of huge numbers of missiles which have never before been fired simultaneously. The Soviets would have to believe that missile accuracy tested in flights across their continent could be duplicated by missiles actually flying over the North Pole, where unique geophysical conditions may drive the missiles off course. Similarly, they would have to believe that the blast and shock waves from the first nuclear warheads to land would not destroy other incoming missiles short of their targets—the problem of "fratricide."

Even if Soviet leaders could assume the total success of an untried attack that can never be tested in advance, they would also have to assume that an American President would simply allow our ICBMs to be destroyed instead of firing them before they were hit—that is, launching them after the Soviet attack has begun. What incentive would a President have, in Soviet calculations, for not using the ICBMs before losing them? Soviet leaders would also have to assume that, even if more than 20 million Americans perished in the short span of a counterforce attack, the President would refuse to retaliate with submarine missiles, bombers, and remaining ICBMs. How could Soviet leaders be sure that their American counterparts would consider such a first strike a "limited" attack, not calling for a response? A minimum of 4000 American strategic warheads would survive a perfect Soviet assault. At least half of the 32 U.S. submarines would be available to strike back after a first strike. Just one submarine, the *Poseidon*, carries 160 independently targetable warheads, each with a yield equivalent to three Hiroshima bombs. That one submarine could inflict untold losses on the Soviet Union.

It seems safe to conclude that national leaders with even the slightest interest in the survival of their citizens and the continuation of their society could not rationally contemplate a first strike. But technology may soon rationalize the irrational. The United States and the Soviet Union are moving ahead with the development and deployment of a complex array of new weapons that potentially pose a first-strike threat to a very significant percentage of the other side's nuclear arsenal. Instead of assessing the real strategic, political, and economic vulnerability of the USSR, our government laments the death of the American strategic superiority. By insisting that the United States is a second-class strategic power, a proposition which has no basis in fact, the administration is elevating world perceptions of Soviet strategic power to undeserved heights, while unnecessarily eroding our own image in the eyes of our allies and our enemies.

The next round of the arms race is not only nonsensical; it could also prove to be profoundly destabilizing. Despite a few interruptions, we have been on a course toward greater and then ultimate instability ever since Hiroshima. At that time a series of technological innovations began to fundamentally alter the way in which we could and should think about war. Because of the enormous destructive power of nuclear weapons, the quest to actively and effectively defend the entire expanse of society became increasingly futile. It was painfully clear, once the Soviets had duplicated American development of the bomb, that both sides lived unavoidably with a "balance of terror." In short, neither side could launch nuclear weapons first because, no matter what the size, timing, or ferocity of an attack, the aggressors could expect a retaliatory, or second, strike that would rain death upon its people and its entire social, military, and industrial structure. This standoff has maintained a precarious but "stable" peace.

Despite the currently impressive U.S. threat, the Soviets need not move their ICBM arsenal into a dangerous launch-on-warning status at the present time. The Soviet leadership knows that a significant portion of its arsenal can still ride out an attack and respond with a lethal barrage. Similarly, the United States knows that significant portions of our

forces can endure a surprise attack and react with overwhelming force. This mutual knowledge has immeasurably
added to stability in times of crisis; and it is this invaluable
sense of stability that could be lost to the complexities of
emerging weaponry. If both nations continue to worship the
false goal of nuclear superiority, weapons systems will emerge
which drastically reduce global security. In the absence of a
mutual nuclear freeze, advances in weapons technology on
each side will threaten the confidence of both sides concerning the survivability of their retaliatory forces. Peace could be
at the mercy of a few minutes of decision making.

The Soviet Union and the United States have been engaged
in programs which will increase the accuracy and destructive
potential of their missiles. For the United States, this process
involves the retrofitting of 300 Minuteman III ICBMs with a
more destructive warhead, the MK-12A. Each of 900 MK-
12A warheads will have twice the accuracy and double the
explosive power of the present Minuteman III warheads. The
Soviet Union could regard them as a substantial threat to the
survivability of their land-base missiles, just as we regard
their SS-18 and other ICBMs as a threat to our land-base
missiles. In fact, compared to the United States, more than
twice as much of Soviet nuclear force is based on land, and
would be vulnerable in theory to a U.S. first-strike attack.

The United States is still developing the MX (Missile Experimental), which is nearing the production stage and could
be deployed as early as 1986. The MX will be the most powerful and accurate missile ever constructed. It combines massive throw-weight with an unmatched guidance system. It is a
highly advanced weapon with at least ten warheads per missile; 200 MX missiles would provide the U.S. with the potential to smash a large portion of Soviet ICBMs in their silos.
The Soviets could conclude that their land-based missiles,
comprising almost 75 percent of the total Soviet strategic arsenal, could fall to a U.S. first strike by the end of this
decade.

The United States is also improving its submarine-based
force with plans to deploy the advanced Trident II subma-
rine-launched missile. In the past, submarine missiles have
been too small and inaccurate to claim effective counterforce
capability. But the new Trident missiles already have substantial counterforce characteristics; they are accurate and
destructive enough to jeopardize military targets. If the

United States continues in the planned deployment of the advanced Trident II missile in 1989, we will have the first survivable submarine force with, at minimum, a plausible capacity for an effective attack on Soviet land-based missiles.

A sea-based threat of this kind raises ominous and complex questions of stability during a crisis. Submarine missiles have far fewer miles to fly, and far shorter trajectories to travel, than ICBMs. Fearing the loss of an overwhelming part of their ICBMs, bombers, and submarines in port, Soviet leaders could be forced to make a decision on launching forces out from underneath the incoming attack within as little as ten minutes.

In the 1960s and 1970s the Soviet Union, relying on somewhat inferior technology, decided to build missiles with larger warheads of up to 25 megatons to offset the fact that the missiles were not coming close enough to their targets. The Soviets are beginning to resolve this problem. Over the past decade, they have made significant strides in refining missile accuracy. The SS-19, the Soviets' newest, most accurate and reliable missile, nearly rivals present American systems. The Russians are modernizing the SS-19 and they are preparing a new ICBM, which will augment their potential to hit American missiles in their silos.

For many years, the Soviets have faced persistent geographical and technical barriers to submarine missile force development, but they have made important headway. A new generation of Soviet submarine missiles now in the development phase could significantly improve the capacity of such missiles to destroy cities in the continental United States. While the Soviet Union is far from matching U.S. submarine technologies at the level of the Trident submarine or the Trident II missile, it is probable that, in the absence of a freeze or other restraints, Soviets submarines will eventually achieve a first-strike potential against American ICBMs.

It may not matter in terms of the risks during a confrontation that a first strike, as we have seen, probably could not be truly effective. What matters is what each side perceives, or thinks the other side perceives. With both superpowers developing more accurate and destructive missiles, a rising sense of mutual vulnerability will breed fear and doubt. If both sides feel that they may have to launch increasingly vulnerable land-based missiles on warning of an approaching attack, we may someday witness a reciprocal recycling of fears between national leaders, with the existence of the industrialized world hanging in the balance. The new weapons of tomorrow could make the costs and casualties of not striking first seem so high that leaders caught in crisis may feel that they have no choice but to shoot first and ask questions later. History could soon parallel the opening of World War I in August 1914, when nobody wanted war, but misperceptions, inflexible mobilization plans, and fear of waiting forced events out of control. The guns of August could become the nuclear missiles of the final world war.

Without a weapons freeze, the long-term view toward the technological horizon is bleak and alarming. Technological advances could make human participation in crisis decisions virtually obsolete. Already both sides depend heavily on computers for such decisions. Given that the flight time of an ICBM from one continent to the other is little more than 30 minutes, satellites, radars, and computers are the only way to collect an encyclopedic array of accurate information about the origin, size, and destination of an apparent attack. There are those who take solace in the rationality of humanity and dismiss scenarios of nuclear war as too awful for any leader to contemplate. But at some point, there might hardly be any time for a genuinely human choice to be made. Someday the computers may dominate the question of whether and how to retaliate. That day may not be distant.

Moreover, weapons systems already deployed have dramatically reduced the span of warning time. The Soviet SS-20 can reach London in less than 15 minutes. The Pershing II missile currently planned for the NATO countries can strike at Moscow just as swiftly. Both countries can fire submarine missiles at special trajectories to avoid detection; and by lying close to shore, the submarines can cut the margin for decision to approximately 15 minutes. Warning times could also be slashed by new systems now under development such as supersonic cruise missiles, or fractional orbital bombardment systems. FOBS whose missiles reach their target by travelling into outerspace and back to earth make detection more difficult.

In the absence of a freeze before the next round in the arms race, a new and volatile mixture of weaponry and apprehension may set the stage for perhaps the tensest period of the nuclear age, a stage on which the war game could be played out and the human drama could be closed out. Inexorably, we may move beyond massive assured destruction to a nuclear psychology that is madder than MAD.. Some of those who agree with this long-term prognosis nonetheless argue that now is not the time to freeze testing and restrict technology, that we should do so later, somewhere down the road, after the construction of certain new weapons which they regard as essential to perfect our deterrent. But there always will be a new weapon to be built, a final frill to be added to our deterrent. Somewhere in this process, the technological advances which make new and modernized weapons destabilizing and dangerous may rob us of any opportuntiy to freeze and then to reduce nuclear arms.

Now more than ever, given the present climate of suspicion, instability and tension in the world, arms control cannot be based on trust. Agreements between adversaries must, in part, be verifiable by what the experts call "national technical means"—electronic and satellite intelligence. Over the past two decades, the advent of satellite technology and the advances in radar have made successful arms control negotiations between the superpowers possible. But the use of independent means of verification depends and will continue to depend on the types of weapons and delivery systems themselves. Missiles, submarines, and bombers are all relatively large and difficult to conceal from the effective, probing eye of a satellite. As we move toward the twenty-first century, however, the nature of delivery systems as well as the weapons themselves, could undermine the potential for verification.

The U.S. sea-launched cruise missile, a pilotless jet aircraft aimed from surface ships and submarines, will complicate verification because its small size makes it so concealable. This missile, which could be equipped with conventional or nuclear explosives, will be capable of flying at very low altitudes and closely following the terrain to evade detection. During the 1980s, the U.S. Navy plans to build as many as 4000 such cruise missiles. Many of them could conceivably be placed on tankers, merchant ships, and other nonmilitary vessels. That possibility, by itself, will reduce the Soviet confidence in any system of verification; meanwhile, Soviet advances in their own cruise missile technology will force the United States to cope with corresponding concerns in later years.

The foreseeable mobility of ICBMs deployed in "deceptive

basing modes" could also undermine verification. The original shell-game plan to disguise MX missiles by shuttling them among multiple underground shelters—in effect, a mass transit system for missiles—was theoretically verifiable because of "cooperative" measures planned by the United States. At intervals, all the shelters would have been opened so Soviet satellites could count the number of missiles actually inside, and verify that only a fraction of the shelters actually contained an MX. This is no assurance that future plans for such systems would incorporate elaborate schemes to aid monitoring by the other side. To freeze now, before verification is insecure, will block the deployment of Soviet or American weapons like the MX and the sea-launched cruise missile. This may represent the only hope to preserve the verifiability, and thus the possibility, of arms control.

We have had opportunities in the past to halt the arms race, and for our shortsightedness we have paid an exorbitant price. In 1955, we conceivably could have agreed to prevent the deployment of any intercontinental missiles, a decision that would have drastically slowed, and perhaps ended, the nuclear weapons competition. In the early 1970s we had the opportunity to stop further testing and deployment of multiple, independently targetable warheads before they revolutionized the strategic balance. That missed possibility opened the way to the impending era of first-strike temptations.

The lasting achievements of the treaty banning most antiballistic missiles demonstrates the wisdom of limiting weapons before they are widely produced and deployed. Once new technology becomes attainable, it acquires a bureaucratic mementum which makes its eventual deployment almost inevitable.

The U.S. and the USSR have never been as strategically equivalent as they are today. Moreover, this rough parity exists in a nuclear environment where neither side has yet acquired an effective first-strike capability, and where verification remains secure. A new arms race will make a shambles of the present balance and the present opportunity for arms control. A decade shadowed by the high-tension brinksmanship of a first-strike world can be avoided. It will require, however, a historic decision to freeze the testing, production, and deployment of nuclear weaponry on both sides.

The United States should move forcefully to propose a mutual and verifiable freeze to the Soviet Union. Such an agreement would offer a profound opportunity for nuclear stability by limiting the emerging threat of counterforce weaponry, and by breaking the impasse that prevents major reductions in current stockpiles of nuclear arms. A freeze on testing of nuclear explosives can inhibit technical improvements in the design and size of warheads, improvements that would refine their accuracy. A freeze on test-firing of new missiles would mean that neither side could develop the unsettling apprehension that the other has acquired a plausible first-strike capability. A freeze on production and deployment would stop the addition of large numbers of warheads, missiles, and bombers to Soviet and American arsenals.

A freeze means that we will not have to run the next round of the arms race. If we do, it will be a different race than the two superpowers have known before. It will continue to be a contest without a finish line where both sides seek to win nuclear superiority but each side always matches the other, stride for stride. The cost of the race will remain expensive; indeed it will become more expensive than ever before. By 1985 the United States will spend more on the military budget than the entire spending of the federal government from the ratification of the Constitution in 1789 until the middle of World War II. But the most fearsome difference will be in the nature of the race itself. As technology rushes ahead, the runners who use it in the race will be increasingly shrouded from each other, their arsenals and intentions more and more unclear. Both may have a sense of mounting threat. This will be a race run in a nuclear twilight, on the edge of a gathering nighttime, where fewer rules can be made or enforced because violations will become less and less visible, and because preparations for aggression will be made in secret and executed with hardly any warning at all. The next round in the arms race, more than any other that has been run before, threatens to become the last chapter in modern history.

7

THE PEOPLE SPEAK AND AMERICA BEGINS TO LISTEN

"The unleashed power of the atom has changed everything save our modes of thinking and we thus drift toward unparalleled catastrophe."

—Albert Einstein

Both of us have been deeply concerned about the issue of nuclear survival throughout our careers in public life. One of us, Edward Kennedy, was 13 years old when the atomic bomb exploded over Hiroshima, the same age as Shigeko Sasamori and Hiroko Harris, whose stories are told in Chapter One. In 1978, returning from a trip to the People's Republic of China, the Kennedy family stopped in Hiroshima and stood at ground zero. Later, at Hiroshima University, that 13-year-old who had since become a United States Senator told the students: "It is impossible to visit Hiroshima without feeling a deep obligation to avoid the holocaust which twice visited Japan. In the novel *Black Rain*, Masuji Ibuse characterized the nuclear explosion as 'More like a jellyfish than a mushroom—writhing and raging as though it might hurl itself on our heads at any moment. It was an envoy of the devil itself, I decided: who else in the whole wide universe would have presumed to summon forth such a

112

monstrosity?' Hiroshima today stands as a living testament to the necessity for progress toward nuclear disarmament; for preventing the spread of nuclear weapons and for progressively reducing their numbers in the few countries that have them today. We must all rededicate ourselves to forestalling the destructive application of nuclear energy, not merely for reasons of strategy but for reasons of humanity. The nuclear arms race of the past thirty years is a tragic story of continuing folly in the face of the lessons of history."

For Mark Hatfield, who was in Hiroshima in 1945, the memories constantly return. This is how the memory seemed on the day when the Kennedy-Hatfield resolution was announced: "I suppose we are all products of our own experiences, which have tremendous impact and influence on our lives. But let me take you back to a particular moment in my life. It was in September of 1945 that I stood in the city of Hiroshima, after the bomb had been dropped and before the rubble had been cleared, while the bodies were still to be retrieved and given proper burial. I could not help but be so totally overwhelmed by the utter and indiscriminate destruction that existed on every hand. Looking in one direction or any other direction in that city, there was nothing but a mass of rubble and the stench of rotting human life. And after that experience, I could say that the bomb had probably saved my life, because we were staging for the operation to invade Japan in a few months. And as we moved into that country to occupy it, it was obvious that we would have suffered a tremendous loss of life in an invasion. But even then, I had a sense of ambivalence about the kind of power that had been unleashed in the world. I wrote home to my parents, who I thought were rather silly sentimentalists to save the letters, but I was very happy that they did, so that I can refer back to my innermost feelings that I had put on paper."

Nearly four decades after Hiroshima and Nagasaki, no other nuclear bombs have been dropped in war. The world survives by the grace of God and a thin margin of good fortune, and it will have a better chance of surviving if the nuclear weapons freeze campaign succeeds in bringing statesmen to their senses about a perilous arms race.

The history of the freeze campaign is the story of an idea that took root in America in the 1980s because the time was right and the country was ready. In 1979 the SALT II Treaty between the United States and the Soviet Union was in trouble in the Senate; in fact, as most knew, the Senate's advice was likely to be "no" and its consent was likely to be withheld. The prospects for ratification of the treaty were poor because of a deepening polarization over strategic policy and a sudden new controversy over Soviet troops in Cuba. In a few months, the treaty simply faded into the background; the Soviet Union invaded Afghanistan, and President Carter decided not even to ask for a Senate vote.

Although SALT II had not yet failed to win ratification in the autumn of 1979, supporters of arms control were discouraged enough to cast about for another way to revive the hope for progress. They began to understand that the SALT process was in collapse because the country had no effective constituency for nuclear arms control, and that there would never be any such constituency without a proposal that people could understand and support. Historically, in the late 1950s and early 1960s, it was public concern over radioactive fallout from the atmosphere which had made it possible for President Kennedy to negotiate the landmark Test-Ban Treaty with the Soviet Union and win its ratification in the Senate. In the late 1960s and the early 1970s, it was public opposition to the Sentinel and Safeguard anti-ballistic missile systems and the futility of such defenses against nuclear attack which persuaded President Nixon to negotiate an ABM treaty; this agreement limited the United States and the Soviet Union to two anti-ballistic missile sites each; only one was ever built in each country. And in 1980 and 1981 it was the intense opposition of farmers and ranchers and the Mormon Church in Utah and Nevada that blocked President Carter's plan to dig up thousands of square miles of western land so that the Pentagon could plant a new supergeneration of ballistic missiles called MX.

In the best tradition of democracy, the nuclear weapons freeze campaign started, not in Washington, but in the grass roots of America. The nationwide movement grew from the seeds of individual concern about the inadequacies of SALT process, the lukewarm popular support it received, and the reluctance of the Senate to ratify even that limited agreement. In the summer of 1979 the American Friends Service Committee adopted a proposal for a "Nuclear Moratorium," which called upon the United States to cease production and deployment of new nuclear weapons for a period of three years; the AFSC felt that the Soviet Union would reciprocate, and that both sides could then proceed to negotiate major reductions in their nuclear arsenals. But the proposal was controversial because of its suggestion that the United States should act unilaterally, without a corresponding commitment to restraint by the Soviet Union.

That same summer, Randall Forsberg, a 38-year-old defense analyst and arms control activist who had worked many years with the Stockholm International Peace Research Institute, took an indefinite leave of absence from her graduate studies at MIT to found the Institute for Defense and Disarmament Studies in Brookline, Massachusetts. Forsberg was born in Alabama but grew up in New York, where her family had moved when she was three so that her father could pursue his career as an actor. An English major at Barnard College in New York City, Forsberg became a defense analyst almost by accident, editing manuscripts at the Stockholm Institute. In 1979, she coauthored a book that became an important resource in the debate over national defense, the Boston Study Group's *The Price of Defense.*

Forsberg hoped that her new institute in Brookline would develop into a respected source of information about Soviet and American military programs, as well as a catalyst for new directions in arms control. Speaking at rallies, teach-ins, and arms control symposia around the country, Forsberg came to understand the need for an initiative that would be not only acceptable to experts, but capable of firing the public imagination. In travels and lectures during the next year, she earned a reputation as a forceful and persuasive advocate for the concept of a comprehensive nuclear weapons freeze under two additional conditions—it would have to be bilateral with the Soviet Union and verifiable by both sides.

At meetings with national peace and church-related organizations in the fall of 1979, activists urged Forsberg to draft a document defining a nuclear weapons freeze and defending its feasibility. In December 1979, after her keynote address in Louisville to Mobilization for Survival, a national coalition of grass-roots antinuclear groups, she agreed to distill the speech for publication; back in Brookline, she produced the first draft of a specific proposal for a comprehensive freeze. In the spring of 1980 she published what has become the founding document of the nuclear weapons freeze movement, "Call to Halt the Nuclear Arms Race." Explaining the commitment that has shaped her career and guided her effort, she says: "As a child, I remember being horrified watching war movies of people killing each other. I see the freeze as the first step toward ending war. The arms race has to stop sometime, somehow, and it seemed to me in 1979 that we had as good a shot in the early 1980s as we ever would, if everyone focused on the same thing."

Among the first arms control experts to endorse Forsberg's call were three faculty colleagues at MIT: Phillip Morrison, who had served in the 1940s in the original Manhattan Project that developed the atomic bomb; George Rathjens, the chief scientist of the Department of Defense in the Eisenhower administration and a specialist in nuclear nonproliferation in the Carter administration; and Bernard Feld, chairman of the Pugwash conferences of scientists and the long-time editor-in-chief of the *Bulletin of Atomic Scientists*.

By summer 1980 the American Friends Service Committee and other national peace and religious organizations, including the Fellowship of Reconciliation, Clergy and Laity Concerned, Sojourners, and Pax Christi, had not only endorsed Forsberg's "Call to Halt the Nuclear Arms Race," but had made it their highest priority.

Simultaneously, the initial stirrings of the new grass-roots movement against the nuclear arms race were being felt in western Massachusetts. They first appeared at the tiny Traprock Peace Center in Deerfield, founded by Randall Kehler and others in 1979 to promote nuclear disarmament and the nonviolent resolution of conflicts. An undergraduate at Harvard in the 1960s, Kehler had left college for a year to teach elementary school in Tanzania. Later, he dropped out of graduate work in education at Stanford to join the anti-Vietnam War movement on the West Coast. In 1973, he returned to Massachusetts and settled in the small town of Colrain on the North River, a few miles from the Vermont border, where he began teaching Spanish in secondary school and doing research on economic and energy issues for the Massachusetts state government and the Cooperative Extension Service of the U.S. Department of Agriculture. Tracking the debate on the SALT II Treaty in Congress in 1979 and drawing on discussions with Sojourners and his interest in a strategic weapons moratorium amendment offered by Mark Hatfield to the SALT Treaty in the Senate, Kehler conceived a political strategy for testing the idea of a comprehensive nuclear weapons freeze in western Massachusetts. In January 1980, with his Traprock friends, he launched a nine-month campaign for a nuclear freeze initiative on the ballot in three state senate districts. The proposal instructed the senators from the area to introduce a resolution in the Massachusetts Senate calling upon the President of the United States to propose to the Soviet Union that both countries adopt an immediate nuclear weapons freeze and transfer the funds saved to civilian use.

In September representatives of more than a dozen organizations working independently to advance the freeze concept met in New York City to assess their progress and prepare a long-term strategy. It was clear that the various local freeze campaigns had touched a sensitive public nerve, and that the time was ripe for a national effort. From this meeting came an ad hoc national strategy committee and a conference planning committee. A Massachusetts businessman attending the meeting, Alan Kay, agreed to donate a small sum to finance the first national conference. After the meeting, Kehler redoubled his efforts in western Massachusetts, saying, "By God, we've got to pull out all the stops and win our initiative in November, or else all the tremendous potential represented by this meeting will never be realized." Concerned about the growing support for the Reagan presidential campaign, and its anti-arms control aura, Kehler was convinced that the only remedy was to demonstrate that solid public support did exist for ending the nuclear arms race; it was there, waiting to be tapped.

Returning to Massachusetts, Kehler shifted the ballot initiative into higher gear, using radio spots, newspaper editorials, television news, and door-to-door campaigning. The endorsement of Silvio Conte, the Congressman from western Massachusetts, was a key development before the election. The freeze was on the ballot in 62 cities and towns in the three districts; the 150,000 voters who turned out approved the freeze by a 3 to 2 margin. The success of the campaign made it a model for others to come, but the result was largely ignored by the press, the Congress, and the new President. In fact, 33 western Massachusetts towns had voted for Ronald

Reagan, and 30 of these had also voted for the freeze. The 1400 people of Colrain, Kehler's hometown, voted two-to-one for the Reagan-Bush ticket and two-to-one for the freeze initiative. President Reagan was confidently announcing a mandate from the people for adding more overkill to the nation's nuclear arsenal, but Kehler and his fellow organizers had a mandate of their own that most pollsters and pundits had missed. The budding freeze campaign was becoming a public antidote against the danger of a new round of the arms race. The movement was evolving into a national force with a common sense solution, and it was attracting the support even of voters who had strongly favored President Reagan.

In March 1981, the National Freeze Campaign held its first annual conference in Washington, D.C.; 16 of 18 town meetings in Vermont had just voted for the freeze. From the meeting came a broad-based National Committee to coordinate policy decisions, a smaller Executive Committee to oversee the creation of a National Freeze Clearinghouse, and a series of task forces in areas such as fund raising, national media, educational materials, international contacts, relations with Congress and the administration, and outreach programs to other organizations and communities. After the conference, statewide efforts accelerated and freeze campaigns leapfrogged from state to state. The Massachusetts legislature endorsed the freeze by nearly unanimous votes of the Senate in May and the House in June; Oregon approved a similar measure a few days later, followed in a few weeks by the New York State Assembly. The legislatures of Connecticut, Maine, Minnesota, Vermont, and Wisconsin soon joined, as did the House of Representatives in Kansas and Iowa and the State Senate in Maryland.

In Oregon, the movement picked up speed early in 1981, when Peter Bergel, a staff assistant to State Representative Wally Priestley of Portland, started writing to Randy Forsberg. Within six months, the legislature had passed a measure offered by Priestley and State Senator Ted Kulongoski of Junction City, calling for a bilateral nuclear weapons freeze; Oregon had become the second state to approve the freeze. Bergel also helped to found a new organization in Salem, Citizen's Action for Lasting Security, which has become an important part of the freeze campaign, not only in Oregon, but nationwide.

At the same time, a separate focus of the nuclear freeze developed in California under the direction of Harold Willens, an executive who had founded Businessmen Against the Vietnam War in the early 1970s. An advocate of controls on both nuclear and conventional forces, Willens had helped establish the Center for Defense Information in Washington, D.C., and the Interfaith Center to Reverse the Arms Race in Pasadena, California. As in Massachusetts, it was grass-roots action that laid the initial groundwork for the California campaign. Inspired by the results of the freeze initiative in western Massachusetts, Jo and Nick Seidita, a housewife and a schoolteacher in Los Angeles, spent many weeks speaking and organizing around the state in 1981. They sought out Willens, who agreed to help with organizing and fundraising. In September 1981 a statewide freeze campaign was officially launched in California with Willens as chairman and Porter Briggs, publisher of *Aquaculture* magazine in Arkansas, as manager. The initial campaign goal was a petition drive to collect the 346,000 signatures needed to put the nuclear freeze issue on the statewide ballot for the November 1982 elections; by April the campaign had already topped 600,000 signatures.

In Washington, D.C., the Nuclear Freeze Foundation focuses on coordinating the grass-roots movement with Congressional interest in the freeze. The foundation offers briefings for members of the Senate and the House and provides liaison for Congress with arms control experts and defense specialists. It is also an information resource about freeze activities in Congress and how they relate to state and local efforts. The foundation's aim is to work closely with the national freeze movement and bolster its effort. It also serves to counter the antifreeze campaign of the Senate and Defense Departments and others in the administration.

Several other groups have made vital contributions to the freeze movement. Physicians for Social Responsibility, founded in 1962, was reactivated in 1980 by Helen Caldicott, an Australian-born pediatrician at Children's Hospital in Boston. For the past two years, under Caldicott as president and Thomas Halsted as director, PSR has mobilized a large number of physicians and other health professionals to make government officials and private citizens face up to the real

consequences of a nuclear attack; Dr. Jack Geiger, Dr.
Howard Hiatt, and other members of PSR have testified before Congress about the massive individual casualty count
and the nationwide health care nightmare that would occur in
such a war. Enrollment in PSR, which supports a nuclear
weapons freeze, has soared from ten members in 1979 to
12,000 in 1982; 6000 additional persons have become financial sponsors, and chapters in 45 states are providing accessible and highly credible sources of information about the
nuclear danger. As a flourishing national organization, the
PSR phenomenon reflects the deepening commitment of scientists and physicians—the men and women who know the most
about the human dimension of nuclear war—to see that it
never happens.

A similar commitment drives the Federation of American
Scientists, which includes 45 Nobel prizewinners in physics,
chemistry, and biology on its board of sponsors. Established
in 1946 by scientists involved in the development of the first
atomic bomb, FAS members today, like their director Jeremy
Stone, see themselves as heirs of the original founders, who
knew too much to be satisfied with doing nothing more than
their scientific work. They know that arms control as well as
nuclear weapons freeze, which the Federation has endorsed,
constitute a task as urgent now as the first race to build
atomic weapons seemed in World War II.

Finally, a new organization called Ground Zero was
formed in 1980 by Roger Molander, who had served on the
National Security Council in the White House from 1974 to
1981. Molander and many of his associates became experts in
arms control and nuclear weapons. Through Ground Zero,
which now has chapters in 140 cities, they are sharing that
expertise with ordinary citizens. Ground Zero is an educational effort, based on the belief that people will do something about the multiplication of nuclear overkill, once they
know enough about the danger. Ground Zero Week, April 19
to 25, 1982, was designed to be for the nuclear arms control
movement what Earth Day is for the environmental movement—confirmation that a new consciousness exists in this
country and will not be denied.

You can find out more about each of these organizations
and their activities and resources by contacting their national
headquarters:

National Freeze Clearinghouse
Nuclear Weapons Freeze Campaign*
414 Lindell Boulevard
St. Louis, Missouri 63108
(314) 533-1169

Nuclear Freeze Foundation
418 C Street, N.E.
Washington, D.C. 20002
(202) 544-2596

Physicians for Social Responsibility
23 Main Street
Watertown, Massachusetts 02172
(617) 924-3468

Federation of American Scientists
307 Massachusetts Avenue, N.E.
Washington, D.C. 20002
(202) 546-3300

Ground Zero
806 15th Street, N.W.
Washington, D.C. 20003
(202) 638-7402

Other organizations have also played an important role in
the growth of the nuclear freeze movement. The Union of
Concerned Scientists has reached millions of Americans nationwide in its campaign to reduce the dangers of nuclear
weapons and nuclear power. The Committee for East-West
Accord and the Committee for National Security focus
concern in Washington on the need to promote national security and nuclear arms control. The Arms Control Association and the Center for Defense Information are important
additional centers of public discussion and education on issues of arms control and national defense.

During the early gestation of the freeze campaign, both authors of this book were working in the Senate to build sup-

*In Appendix C, you will find a complete list of all the local chap-
ters of this organization.

port for the SALT II Treaty. The eclipse of the treaty, coupled with the election of President Reagan in November 1980 on a platform of increased spending for weapons like the B-1 bomber and M-X missile, enhanced our concern about the risk of nuclear war and the threat implicit in yet another round of the arms race. We heard from increasing numbers of citizens anxious about the nuclear future, including scientists and religious leaders, workers and businessmen, pupils and teachers, veterans of the armed forces, and even government officials. All of them were troubled by the apparent readiness of the Kremlin and the White House to countenance policies of increasing confrontation and nuclear brinkmanship. Preoccupied in the first half of 1981 with the Reagan tax and budget proposals and the state of the economy, Congress as a whole was not yet attuned to the gathering public mood. But the year-long debate over the defense buildup, particularly the controversy over the M-X missile and its possible first-strike capability, slowly sensitized the House and the Senate to the nuclear question. Attention mounted when enormous mass demonstrations erupted in Amsterdam, Bonn, London, and other cities in Western Europe over the Reagan administration's failure to pursue nuclear arms control in Europe while proceeding with the planned European deployment of U.S. cruise missiles and Pershing II missiles. President Reagan and Secretary of State Alexander Haig spoke unguardedly of the possibility of fighting a limited nuclear war and of the desirability of firing a nuclear warning shot in the event of a Soviet nonnuclear attack on NATO. Demonstrations intensified in Europe and former Under Secretary of State George Ball, a noted observer of U.S.-European relations since World War II, remarked: "Though the Administration's' statements and policies may not scare the Soviets, they certainly frighten our friends. Our European allies are more and more questioning the leadership of a nation whose government seems addicted to a rhetoric even more bellicose than the Soviets'."

Bowing to reality, President Reagan in November 1981 offered to begin a new round of negotiations on nuclear arms control by suggesting a "zero option" plan for Euromissiles. Under this idea, the Russians would dismantle existing intermediate-range missiles based in the Soviet Union and targeted against Western Europe. The plan would also cover Soviet missiles pointed against China, in order to prevent the Russians, the administration said, from turning them around and pointing them against our European allies. In return, NATO would withdraw its plan to begin the deployment of intermediate-range missiles in Western Europe capable of hitting the Soviet Union. But on December 13, 1981, the Soviet-inspired martial law regime was imposed on Poland, and dissolved whatever slim hope there was for any early U.S.-Soviet arms agreement.

Events like these rapidly raised the level of public apprehension in the United States, and the nuclear freeze movement quickly took root in communities across the country. During the adjournment of Congress for the Christmas holidays at the end of 1981, both of the authors were struck by the compelling public feeling for the freeze in Oregon and Massachusetts and by its range of support among constituents of every age, faith, race, philosophy, and sex. A sleeping giant of public opinion had suddenly awakened, including not only peace activists, but a broad new constituency reflecting America as a whole; in the language of nuclear physics, it seemed that the freeze movement had reached the critical mass needed to start a powerful public reaction. Grandparents asked to meet with us, and the issues they wanted to discuss were not only Social Security and the Reagan budget cuts, but their worry that nuclear war was coming in the lifetime of their grandchildren. We heard about a survey of elementary and secondary school students by a task force of the American Psychiatric Association, which found that the imminent threat of nuclear annihilation had penetrated deeply into the consciousness of the students; the great majority did not believe that they or their city or their country could survive a nuclear attack. We met large numbers of people deeply concerned about the failure of their government to perceive what so many of them instinctively understand: that the United States and the Soviet Union already have more than enough nuclear power to destroy each other, even after suffering a first nuclear strike; that each side will inevitably match the other's nuclear buildup and raise the ante higher; and that the result of this overheated nuclear poker game may be a nuclear war that could incinerate most Americans and most Russians as well.

As we traveled in our two states, we heard from people at

every stop who knew about the nuclear freeze proposal and wanted us to support it. "Why not?" they asked. We found that question difficult to answer then, just as many of our colleagues in the Senate and the House of Representatives are finding it difficult to answer now. By the time the Senate convened again at the end of January 1982, we were convinced that a new arms control initiative was needed to offer leadership in Congress and respond to the growing public concern. We asked our staffs to consider arms control alternatives and review them not only with the wide spectrum of defense and foreign policy experts who had advised us over the years, but also with leaders of the nuclear freeze campaign. Out of the array of alternatives, the nuclear freeze proposal showed through with clarity and appeal. Citizens across the country were already raising its banner. Many, although not all, of the experts we consulted said they could support a freeze, including former Under Secretary of State George Ball, retired Chief of Naval Development Admiral Thomas Davies, onetime Deputy CIA Director Herbert Scoville, John Steinbruner of the Brookings Institution, Jeremy Stone of the Federation of American Scientists, and former arms control negotiator Paul Warnke. These authorities, with decades of combined experience in national defense and arms control, allayed doubts raised by other experts and developed a convincing case that the freeze was a practical and verifiable proposal worth trying, and that it might well be the idea with the best chance of success in negotiations with the Soviets. Links with the grass-roots freeze movement came through Christopher Paine of the Federation of American Scientists. As a research fellow at the Council on Economic Priorities in New York in 1979, Paine had participated in the early drafting of the freeze initiative.

After consultation with both the experts and freeze leaders, a proposal was drawn up parallel to the terms of the Forsberg-Kehler initiative in Massachusetts and the Willens effort in California; on March 10, 1982, the Kennedy-Hatfield resolution was introduced in the Senate and an identical measure was offered in the House of Representatives by Edward Markey and Silvio Conte of Massachusetts and Jonathan Bingham of New York. At this writing, the resolution has the sponsorship of 24 members of the Senate and 166 members of the House of Representatives.

The freeze movement was also registering impressive gains

outside the Congress. In addition to the ballot initiatives, town meetings, and actions by state legislatures, hundreds of local groups and over 60 national groups had supported the freeze, including religious, environmental, women's, minority, and other organizations. The National Nuclear Weapons Freeze Campaign in St. Louis had organized in 43 states and 279 congressional districts, and planned to organize in all the remaining states and districts. As Randy Kehler, the campaign's national coordinator, put it, "Because the bilateral freeze is so inherently clear and comprehensible, because it make so much common sense, it is winning the support of a wide spectrum of American people."

That the American people have found an effective way to insist on arms control is evident from the public support which continues to roll in. John Smith, the Mayor of Prichard, Alabama, and a member of the Alabama Conference of Black Mayors, says: "We have come to a civilized position as a nation, and to continue on this course of nuclear buildup is senseless." Like previous powerful and popular movements in American history, the freeze campaign is exerting an impact on national and local policies and politics and will have even greater impact in the future because of the effective way in which local, state, and congressional initiatives are reinforcing each other; the emerging partnership between Congress and grass-roots supporters of the freeze is enhancing its impact and building a popular majority that Congress and the Reagan administration will find increasingly difficult to resist. By April 1982 the freeze initiative had already obliged the administration to accelerate its Strategic Arms Reduction Talks (START) schedule and retreat from its rhetoric about waging limited nuclear wars.

In reaction to the movement's initial success, competing arms control resolutions were introduced in Congress in an effort to derail the Kennedy-Hatfield resolution. Some alternatives embrace the Reagan call for the beginning of START negotiations. Others, such as the Jackson-Warner resolution, introduced in the Senate on March 30, 1982, by Senators Henry Jackson of Washington and John Warner of Virginia and in the House by Congressman William Carney of Hauppauge, New York, pretend to support a freeze while tacitly embracing a nuclear arms buildup. Endorsed by President Reagan, the Jackson-Warner resolution is being used as a thin disguise for the goal of those bent on restoring American nuclear superiority over the Soviet Union. Most citizens realize that any such plan is a brand of nuclear nostalgia dangerous to the country's health. The innate strength of the freeze initiative is the public's willingness to accept American-Soviet nuclear parity in the interest of nuclear survival, rather than engage in a quixotic search for superiority that could end in annihilation. They see a freeze as the critical first step toward recovering U.S.-Soviet sanity in the nuclear age and avoiding the "unparalleled catastrophe" that Albert Einstein foresaw.

Another vital element in the freeze movement has been the early and dedicated advocacy by religious leaders of all faiths. More than 30 prominent Catholic bishops have now endorsed the Kennedy-Hatfield resolution, including Archbishop James Hickey of Washington, D.C., Archbishop John Quinn of San Francisco, and Archbishop Raymond Hunthausen of Seattle. Bishop James Armstrong, President of the National Council of Churches, Reverend Billy Graham, and the leaders of Protestant denominations have given their support. The resolution has also been endorsed by Rabbi Alexander Schindler, President of the Union of American Hebrew Congregations, by Rabbi Walter Wurzburger, President of the Synagogue Council of America, and by other Reform, Conservative, and Orthodox Jewish leaders. The comment of Bishop Roger Mahony of Stockton, California, typifies the moral dimension of the freeze: "Our future as American peoples, as Soviet peoples, as the human race on this planet, demands that we make a moral 'about-face' on the nuclear arms race." Rabbi Schindler says, "The nuclear arms race is emerging as the central moral issue of our day." Rabbi Wurzburger, who survived the Nazi Holocaust in World War II, states: "It is my moral responsibility to raise my voice against policies that may be responsible for our drifting into another nuclear holocaust, which would spell the doom of all of mankind." Bishop Armstrong has observed: "There seems to be a quickening conscience, perhaps belated, across the religious and moral community of humankind, that is responding to the urgent challenge of this hour."

After months of initial skepticism, the nuclear weapons freeze campaign is also gaining adherents among those experienced in arms control, national defense, military intelligence, and foreign policy; supporters range from former Secretaries of State Edmund Muskie and Dean Rusk to former Secretary of Defense Clark Clifford and former CIA

Director William Colby. Three former Ambassadors to the Soviet Union, W. Averell Harriman, George Kennan, and Thomas Watson, have endorsed the freeze; so have General James Gavin and Admiral Noel Gaylor, as have William Foster and Gerard Smith, former Directors of the U.S. Arms Control and Disarmament Agency and U.S. negotiators of the SALT Treaty and the Nuclear Nonproliferation Treaty. Support from these experts effectively rebuts the claim of Secretary of State Alexander Haig that the Kennedy-Hatfield resolution is bad defense policy, bad arms control policy, and bad foreign policy. Admiral Davies states, "The Kennedy-Hatfield Resolution [is] the only rational approach to nuclear weapons. I believe it to be in the national security interest of the United States." Scoville adds: "The key elements of any freeze or reduction agreement that might be negotiated can be adequately verified without a requirement for intrusive and unacceptable procedures. A freeze on the testing, production and deployment of nuclear weapons, leading to deep reductions, as expressed in the Kennedy-Hatfield Resolution, is a sound arms control measure which can lead to greater security for all peoples." George Ball, Under Secretary of State in the Johnson administration, endorsed the freeze in these words: "The Kennedy-Hatfield Resolution provides a sensible alternative to continuing the arms race to the point where the advent of increasingly complex and elaborate new weapons systems will close off our last clear chance for effective negotiation."

Some critics resist the Kennedy-Hatfield resolution because they distrust the intrusion of democracy into sensitive issues of national security; they are reluctant to invite the public into debates where experts usually tread. But try as they may, no professional elite can long maintain a monopoly over the ultimate issue of personal survival for 200 million Americans and their families. The nuclear version of the medieval question How many angels can dance on the head of a pin? is: Precisely how high can the United States and the Soviet Union make each other's radioactive rubble bounce? People already know the answer to that question: The Soviets can make our rubble bounce all the way from Maine to California, and we can make theirs bounce from Moscow to Vladivostok. The Soviet people may not have the right or the power to speak out or to move their totalitarian rulers; but the American people suffer no similar restraint. The strength of democracy in the United States is that men and women can catch the attention of their government and demand that it respond. The nuclear freeze movement and the Kennedy-Hatfield resolution are gaining currency in the American marketplace of ideas because of their clarity and their irrefutable logic that the arms race can be stopped and must be stopped.

8

THE CASE FOR A FREEZE

"It is time to examine our attitude toward peace itself. Too many of us think it is impossible. But that is a dangerous, defeatist belief. It leads to the conclusion that war is inevitable—that mankind is doomed—that we are gripped by forces we cannot control."

—John F. Kennedy
American University
June 1963

In 1963 when President Kennedy, in a commencement address at American University, proposed high-level negotiations with the Soviet Union on the issue of nuclear testing, he was trying in a single but sensible stroke to break a deadlock that had lasted for years. He had dismissed the counsel of some advisers that his offer would be perceived as American weakness. He had listened with disbelief to the argument that the rest of the details had to be worked out before we could ask the Soviet Union to agree to the general principle of an atmospheric test ban. After his address, in the remarkably short span of two months, the remaining details were disposed of and the Test-Ban Treaty of 1963 was signed.

Today there are some officials who, like their counterparts two decades ago, believe that a freeze followed by major reductions in nuclear arsenals is improbable and who argue, in effect, that peace is also impossible. Too many defense ex-

perts who have grown up with the arms race have become
accustomed to guiding it. The agreements negotiated in
SALT I and SALT II have not prevented steadily higher levels of weaponry. As Senators, we supported SALT II because
we thought the country and the world would be better off
with it than without it. It offered a number of limits on nuclear weaponry; without it, there would have been no limits
at all on Soviet and American buildups. But in fact, the
SALT II Treaty, which was never put before the Senate for a
ratification vote, was mostly a means of setting down rules
for limiting the arms buildup, instead of stopping the arms
race and then reversing it.

The SALT process has failed to deal with critical technological advances in weapons and continuing increases in the
number of warheads. In 1960 the United States and the Soviet Union together had 6500 strategic nuclear warheads; today they have 17000. By 1985, when the SALT II Treaty
would have been due to expire, there would have been somewhere between 22,500 and 24,400 such warheads. Though
the treaty was the product of long, hard work against the
background of stiffening political resistance to arms control,
it may have been the best that could be achieved at the time,
at least in domestic terms. But the effort to conciliate the political opposition largely failed. Some critics who originally
wanted no treaty at all charged that the treaty did not do
enough. Many advocates of arms control agreed, but nonetheless argued the comparative advantage of the SALT II
limits.

The weakness of the SALT process in addressing technological breakthroughs has plagued efforts at arms control for
the past decade. The first SALT agreement ignored the advance called MIRV, multiple independently targetable reentry
vehicles, which meant that a single ballistic missile could
carry several warheads, each aimed at a seperate enemy city
or military installation and each sufficient to obliterate it.
Many experts felt that SALT did too little to stop the qualitative arms race and restrain ongoing scientific revolution in
weaponry.

In the 1980s, technology has marched on. Guidance systems have become increasingly and exquisitely accurate; a
missile may now be able to fly 5000 miles and land within a
few hundred feet of the intended target. But exquisitely accurate land-based missiles may also be vulnerable to the other

side's exquisitely accurate missiles. Even in a decade governed by SALT II, both sides could pass beyond the "first-strike" threshold, where either side might assume that it had first-strike capability and first-strike vulnerability simultaneously. The inexorable development of nuclear technology is heading inevitably to a world bristling with hair-trigger nuclear missiles and governed by a "use them or lose them" nuclear psychology. Like sulfur coating a matchstick, the layering of nuclear technology on top of other disputes could erupt in nuclear war any time Americans and Soviets rub each other the wrong way.

Once this strategic Rubicon has been crossed, the possibility of accidental war will rise to an even more dangerous level. On 147 occasions within the past 20 months, U.S. computer malfunctions have signaled a Soviet strategic attack. Four of the incidents were severe enough so that orders were issued to move our strategic forces to a higher state of alert. Once, a mistake caused by a programming error flashed a warning of a Soviet submarine attack. According to the Pentagon, it took six minutes for U.S. command authorities to make a positive identification of the mistake; in a few minutes more, if there had been no mistake, a fusillade of Soviet submarine missiles would have struck our coastal cities. On another occasion, a false signal was flashed from satellites that mistook the rising of the moon for the launching of Soviet missiles.

Some defense analysts behave as if the purpose of arms control is, at most, permanent management of the arms race. But it is unlikely that it can be managed forever and more likely that it will finally manage to destroy much of civilization forever. A nuclear freeze, followed by reductions, is not the only avenue to arms control, but it is the only idea which can stop the spiral of nuclear arms development without the self-defeating delays of endless negotiation over what constitutes equality. In a matter of months, the two superpowers, assuming their goodwill, could reasonably work out verification procedures for a freeze. The former Chief of Naval Development, Admiral Thomas Davies, says:

> Now the virtue of the freeze is to prevent the continued increase of weaponry and the worsening of the situation during a prolonged negotiation. In fact, the history of our negotiations [for arms re-

ductions shows] that they are lengthy and difficult, and during that time there is always a great increase in the number of warheads deployed. So I would say that the freeze is the only practical way to go at that problem.

To freeze first and then negotiate reductions makes sense on many levels. It recognizes the urgency of taking a step that is as simple as it is practical, and that is more feasible now than it has ever been before, because both sides are so nearly equivalent in their arsenals of annihilation.

The freeze agreement would be a firebreak, encircling and containing a weapons race threatening to break out of control. Once armaments and technological advances are stopped at present levels, the two superpowers can negotiate phased and balanced reductions. The Kennedy-Hatfield resolution calls for such reductions "through annual percentages or equally effective means." George Kennan, our former Ambassador to the Soviet Union and our foremost expert on that country, and Admiral Hyman G. Rickover, Director of Naval Nuclear Propulsion under seven Presidents, have argued eloquently and compellingly for deep cuts of at least 50 percent in the nuclear armories of both sides. These cuts could be achieved by the end of this decade, if we mutually agree to reasonable reductions of 7 percent a year. This is the approach proposed in the Kennedy-Hatfield resolution, and suggested by the Senate Committee on Foreign Relations in 1979, which sought sustained major reductions from SALT II ceilings on weaponry.

As the process of reductions moves along, it will be in the interests of both the United States and the Soviet Union to direct their reductions to vulnerable land-based missiles that also provide particularly rapid and precise offensive capability: weapons that could seriously unbalance the basic retaliatory equation which yields mutual deterrence. In short, a freeze on nuclear weapons followed by reductions from their current levels can strengthen deterrence as the purpose of our defense, diminish the risk of accidental nuclear war, and curtail the incentives for the hair-trigger use of nuclear weapons during an escalating crisis.

A freeze will enhance, not reduce, our overall security, because it will prevent the development of more powerful Soviet rockets and block their further deployment of existing weapons. A freeze will prevent one side from perfecting its capacity for a first strike against the other by prohibiting the testing and production of such weapons; the result will be a substantial reduction in the fear of a U.S. or Soviet preemptive attack.

A freeze will also help to strengthen our economy and other areas of our national defense, both of which have heavily suffered from neglect and from the cost of this nuclear buildup. The $90 billion that a freeze alone could save in the next five years could be spent on conventional defenses and domestic priorities. In fact, the strategic arms race is crippling our capacity to meet human needs. We are cutting immunization for children in order to finance the weapons that may someday kill them. Every new shelter for a missile means more spending, a bigger deficit, and higher interest rates, but fewer homes for families. Every new warhead guidance system that can read enemy defenses means there will be more schools where more students will never learn to read. Every new escalation that could mean death at an early age across the earth also darkens the golden years of senior citizens who rely on Social Security, Medicare, and Medicaid, all of which are in danger from cutbacks due to the budget crisis.

The nuclear buildup is an extremely important aspect of the current economic distress. The B-1 bomber alone will cost more than all the job training programs enacted by Congress in the past 20 years. In short, the two greatest issues of our time—the prosperity of the economy and the probability of survival in the nuclear age—are inextricably intertwined. Not only could a freeze save at least $18 billion annually; negotiated reductions could save billions more. A process of mutual nuclear restraint is a needed defense against the prospect of endless budget deficits.

As we have noted, some of the savings from a freeze can be reallocated to improve the readiness and the reliability of our conventional forces. But just as important, when the total burden of military expenditures on the budget is lessened, we will have the resources for the revitalization of our industries and the restoration of America's competitive position in the markets of the world. We will have the funds to develop, and share, alternative energy sources. These tasks are at the heart of the great national security challenges of the 1980s; they are the central arena of testing for the United States, which cannot endure as an insecure or failing economy amid international economic disarray and deprivation.

An eloquent warning of the costs of the arms race came three decades ago from the leader of Republican conservatism. This is what Senator Robert Taft of Ohio said in 1951:

> No nation can be constantly prepared to undertake a full-scale war at any moment and still hope to maintain any of the other purposes in which people are interested and for which nations are founded. In short, there is a definite limit to what a government can spend in time of peace and still maintain a free economy, without inflation and with at least some elements of progress in standards of living and in education, welfare, housing, health and other activities in which people are vitally interested. In my opinion, we are completely able to defend the United States itself. The one great danger we face is that we may overcommit ourselves in this battle against Russia. Let me say that no one is more determined to resist the Communist aggression in the world than I am, but we cannot afford to destroy at home the very liberty which we must sell to the rest of the world as the basis for progress and happiness. In short, a war against Communism in the world must finally be won in the minds of men.

The costs and dangers of the arms race are not new to this administration or to this budgetary crisis. Since World War II, with occasional exceptions, we have paid an accelerating price to prepare for World War III. In 1982 the economic burden of the effort weighs heavier and heavier upon Americans and Soviets alike. President Reagan has observed of the Soviet Union: "Their great military build-up . . . at the expense of the denial of consumer goods . . . has now left them on a very narrow edge." But it is not the adversary alone that now suffers from major economic difficulty. There is no question that if we continue to run an expensive, escalating arms race, we run the risk of Sovietizing our own economy. Investment capital has been drained by the crunching combination of massive increases in military spending, massive deficits, and the resulting scarcity of credit. When resources and strategic materials shortages are factored into the equation, unprecedented military spending may make it impossible for our society ever to return to its previous peaks of prosperity.

We must start retooling now for the future economic character of states from Oregon to Massachusetts, and Michigan to Louisiana. We cannot afford to imitate our adversary by limiting economic progress so that strategic military spending can multiply, vacuuming up every kind of resource. Generally our government has sought to budget federal dollars in ways that leverage private capital formation, jobs and thriving communities; but excessive defense spending actually means more, not less, unemployment. The military has the least multiplier effect of any dollar we spend, while and the highest multiplier comes from a dollar spent on preventive medicine and health. Strategic spending is capital intensive, not labor intensive. Every billion dollars that we spend on the MX missile program will hire 17,000 people, while the same $1 billion could hire 48,000 hospital workers or 65,000 people in the building trades, or 77,000 teachers, police officers, and firefighters.

Few will deny the costs of the arms race in economic and human terms. Instead, opposition to a nuclear freeze, followed by reductions, has focused on military and technical issues. There are certain experts who claim, in effect, that the freeze is a nice but impractical idea. They resist the notion that an issue which was formerly the exclusive province of a professional elite has now become a matter of public debate and intensifying citizen concern. Of course, the management of the nuclear arms race since 1945 has not been a model of success. One argument which freeze opponents are raising now—that the issue is too complex and too important to be left to the people—echoes the argument of an earlier generation that the popular effort to end the Vietnam war was a mistake, or the parallel argument of 1982 that American policy in El Salvador and Central America should be decided in secret.

A number of other analysts and former officials who decry the present arms control stalemate regard the freeze as nothing more than a popular movement which may be beneficial in pressuring the administration, but which does not make sense as national policy because, they say, our strategic forces are not equal to those of the Soviet Union. In fact, there are many experts who favor the Kennedy-Hatfield resolution, ranging from former Secretaries of State and Defense to former CIA executives to America's most capable scientists. There is not a single sensible military or diplomatic official who would trade our strategic forces for the Soviet arsenal. At the present time, the United States is fully capable of defending itself by retaliating fully against any Soviet nuclear attack. America is secure today, and a freeze will preserve that security for the future. Despite all the talk of a "window of vulnerability," this nation and the Soviet Union are at approximate equivalence in strategic nuclear power. In the event of an immediate freeze, we would have 9400 available strategic nuclear warheads and the Soviets would have 7500. Even if a Soviet first strike destroyed all American land-based missiles, we would still have a retaliatory capacity of at least 4000 warheads at sea and in the air. Even congressional testimony from military experts makes reference to the "rough parity" between the two countries. The Defense Department's military posture statement last year stated explicitly that a condition of parity continues to prevail. The current nuclear balance is relatively stable; deterrence still works. By freezing now, we would avoid an age of perceived first-strike threats in which the Soviets would face their own window of vulnerability and which could tempt either side to launch a preemptive strike. And it is that new arms race, not the present situation, which could irrevocably shatter the present balance.

We stand now at a unique moment in the history of the nuclear age where a freeze can work and must be tried. Rather than a window of vulnerability, we now have a window of opportunity for arms control. That window could be slammed shut in the coming years. It is no longer merely enough to call for reductions in nuclear weaponry without calling for a freeze as a first step, and as the only way to keep the window of opportunity open. Critics charge that the Soviets would have no incentive to reduce their arsenals after a freeze. They call for building new systems in order to pile up bargaining chips for negotiations with the Kremlin. But in the past, the arms race has been needlessly perpetuated by this bargaining-chip theory, because both sides feel forced to match new and threatening developments with their own. MIRVs, multiple independent warheads, were defended as a bargaining chip during the SALT I talks. So the United States continued to deploy them and then we were told that they were too important to bargain away.

In contrast, after a freeze both sides will have a vested interest in reductions, since they will still be saddled with weapons which do not add to their security or the effectiveness of their deterrent, which detract from the overall stability of the nuclear balance, and which they can no longer work to perfect. For those whose real aim is a new buildup, the rationale that we need reductions, but not a freeze, is merely a rationalization for amassing the B-1, the M-X, and other new strategic weapons while engaging in protracted negotiations with the Soviets. Frankly, often during negotiations, the United States and the Soviet Union have behaved like fevered patients whose temperature rises from 103 to 104 degrees and who think they're getting better because they're getting sicker at a slower rate.

Past agreements have also been defective because they have not prevented impending leaps in the sophistication of weaponry. Thus the Vladivostok accord and the SALT II Treaty permitted the development of cruise missiles. The military planners saw the loophole and proceeded to rush through it with a weapons system in which they had previously shown only minimum interest. Where there is a loophole, it will almost certainly be exploited. Where a system is permitted, it will be pursued; otherwise, the thinking goes, the adversary will gain an advantage. A comprehensive freeze already in place during reduction talks would plug past loopholes and prevent future ones for the simple reason that it would impose a general moratorium on any and all additions to nuclear arsenals.

Critics of the freeze next suggest that it would leave the United States behind the Soviets in nuclear weaponry in Europe. Officials in the Reagan Administration have presented varying statistics to prove this proposition, citing an inferiority ranging between three-to-one and six-to-one. But such critics exaggerate the facts and distort the true situation in Europe, where the United States, according to the authoritative International Institute for Strategic Studies, has 1,168 available warheads and the Soviets have 2,004. With such numbers each nation has enough to blow up the continent many times over. In any event, the Kennedy-Hatfield resolution rejects a freeze in Europe alone. We are calling for a global freeze. In case of a Soviet nuclear attack on NATO, the United States could call on its entire nuclear arsenal to respond. For the administration to suggest that it no longer relies on this option would signal a major and destabilizing change under which Europe would no longer enjoy the protection of America's nuclear umbrella.

The real and present danger to the NATO alliance, by the estimate of former Under Secretary of State George Ball, is the uncertain and unclear attitude of the United States with respect to the nuclear issue. The sense of apprehension in Europe has been amplified by American discussion of limited nuclear war and nuclear warning shots and by American insistence on the neutron bomb, a malignant scientific breakthrough designed to destroy people through, "enhanced radiation" while minimizing damage to buildings and equipment. Campaigns for unilateral European disarmament gain strength when Washington sounds casual about nuclear conflict and seems uninterested in arms control or unable to achieve progress. Given this record, it is "grotesque," in Secretary Ball's phrase, for the administration to suggest that the Kennedy-Hatfield freeze will undermine the American position in Europe. To the contrary, it can reassure the Europeans that this nation is finally being serious about reducing the risk of accelerating nuclear competition.

Other critics of the resolution have focused on the question of verification. The Kennedy-Hatfield resolution specifically calls for a verifiable freeze. What cannot be verified will not be frozen. But there are many experts who agree that a freeze is largely and sufficiently verifiable. We can have high confidence that one critical aspect of the freeze, deployment, can be verified through "national technical means"—that is, satellites and listening posts equipped with sensors—and through data exchange and restrictions on concealment. A second critical aspect of the freeze, testing, can also be verified by such means together with unmanned seismic stations and opportunities for on-site inspection—both of which the Soviets have already acccepted in principle in the recent negotiations for a Comprehensive Test Ban Treaty. In the past, the United States has regarded such measures as fully adequate for verifying SALT restrictions on deployment and limits on nuclear weapons testing, and they would be fully adequate for verifying these aspects of a nuclear weapons freeze.

A freeze on production of nuclear weapons may be harder to verify, but our intelligence is so well developed, according to former Under Secretary of Defense William Perry, that we have been able to "monitor Soviet activity at the design bureaus and production plants well enough so that we have been able to predict every ICBM before it began its tests." It may be that some form of on-site inspection will be necessary to closely verify production and to check certain limited aspects of testing. To presume that the Soviets will not permit any such inspection overlooks the record of the Comprehensive Test-Ban Treaty negotiations, now postponed by the Reagan administration, where the Soviets have agreed to the principle of on-site verification.

Even areas where there may be verification problems, such as some areas of production, do not present serious difficulties, since verification in other areas would assure overall enforcement of the freeze. Indeed, Herbert Scoville, onetime Deputy Director of the CIA, contends that a freeze is *easier* to verify than a treaty like SALT I or SALT II. Such treaties contain complicated limits on numbers and modifications of missiles and planes; to detect a violation requires continuing and exact measurements of a vast array of possible and prohibited activity. With a freeze, however, a violation would be known if the adversary did anything new at all. And even the one-for-one replacement that would be permitted by a freeze could be verified with high confidence.

We are also told by critics that a freeze will interfere with arms control negotiations now planned or underway. But as we have seen, it could be years before any overall agreement is concluded. Meanwhile a comprehensive freeze can break the fever of the arms race and bring the thermonuclear temperature down. It can also contribute to progress on the formidable problem of nuclear proliferation, the spread of the bomb to other nations, including unstable regimes in the Third World. American and Soviet appeals against such proliferation tend to fall on cynical ears so long as our own nuclear production moves ahead. A freeze can draw a line not only across the arms race, but across the attitudes of the world. It would give the superpowers the moral authority to deal with the gathering disaster of proliferation. It would deprive aspiring nuclear powers of the too ready excuse that they have every right to acquire the bomb so long as we are striving to augment our own massive arsenals.

The Indian nuclear explosion in 1974 forcefully reminded the world of the deadly threat of proliferation. Pakistan has reacted predictably by trying to catch up with India. We now have an arms race in the subcontinent. Where one nation becomes a nuclear power, however modest, neighboring states feel driven to get bombs of their own; this process is globalizing the deadly logic of nuclear threat and counterthreat. And this, in turn, could set off a nuclear confrontation between the United States and the Soviet Union.

Expanding numbers of nuclear weapons around the world could encourage terrorism in the form of nuclear blackmail. The possible scenarios are chilling. Suppose that, Libya, long frustrated in the quest for a nuclear bomb of its own, receives a gift from Pakistan as an act of Islamic solidarity. Colonel Qadhafi then brandishes the bomb against the state of Israel, which he is sworn to destroy. The crisis escalates and engages Qadhafi's Soviet allies and Israel's American allies; there is a regional and then a global nuclear catastrophe.

A credible and effective strategy to prevent such nightmares depends on a number of mutually reinforcing steps. We must strengthen international nuclear safeguards against the diversion of nuclear materials from peaceful to military uses. We must restrain reckless commerce in nuclear energy, by prohibiting the transfer of plutonium reprocessing and uranium enrichment equipment and technology, and by insisting on control of spent nuclear fuel. We must seek more nuclear weapons-free zones such as the one in Latin America.

The key to all of these developments is greater adherence to the current Nuclear Nonproliferation Treaty. A freeze, followed by reductions, can promote that. It is exactly what the treaty itself calls for. By embarking on such a course, the United States and the Soviets can prove that at last, they are observing their pledge under Article VI of the treaty:

> Each of the parties . . . undertakes to pursue negotiations in good faith on effective measures relating to cessation of the nuclear arms race at an early date and to nuclear disarmament, and on a treaty on general and complete disarmament under strict and effective international control.

In effect, a freeze would also be a comprehensive test ban between the superpowers. They could then move to expand it into more formal sanctions against all nuclear tests or explosions.

Finally, some critics suggest that a freeze proposal will be dismissed outright by the Soviet Union. They point to the Soviet rejection of the so-called "deep cuts" suddenly proposed by the Carter administration in 1977. In fact, that experience argues for the more modulated, less complicated strategy of an initial freeze followed by negotiated reductions. The 1977 proposal was highly specific; it asked for agreement to detailed cuts before agreement to the principle of deep cuts. After analyzing the details, Soviet leaders almost certainly interpreted the proposal as locking them into a position of nuclear inferiority. A freeze today would mean a more nearly equivalent balance. In any event, the possibility of rejection by the Soviets is hardly an argument against the desirability of trying for a freeze. If there is any case in history where the imperative of bold initiative applies, it is the nuclear arms race. In the search for arms control, nothing ventured is truly nothing gained, and perhaps in the end, everything truly lost.

In reality, much of the attack on the freeze resolution is a disguise for a different and more unsettling position. The 1983 budget proposal asks for funds to "successfully fight either conventional or nuclear war." This is the first time that any budget proposal has ever said any such thing. We must continue to insist that the American purpose is to deter a nuclear exchange, not to fight one. We must reject the concept of a limited nuclear battle. Admiral Noel Gayler, former Director of the National Security Agency, has acidly dismissed the musings of the limited war theorists: "I have no confidence in the imaginary situations and chess games that a certain school of analysts dreams up. Real war is not like these complicated tit-for-tat imaginings. There is little knowledge of what's going on, and less communication. There is blood and terror and agony, and these theorists propose to deal with a war a thousand times more terrible than any we have ever seen, in some bloodless, analytic fashion. I say that's nonsense. We deceive ourselves, and we deceive our opponent into believing we have aggressive intentions that we do not have." Indeed that is the danger: someday the nuclear war-game theorists may actually find themselves playing the game for real.

The fascination of some experts and politicians with such games, or their attachment to traditional approaches to arms control, has spurred a constant effort to find some simple argument, any simple argument, to dismiss or deflect the freeze proposal. When the critics come to admit, as former Secretary of Defense Harold Brown recently did, that a complete freeze "if immediately and fully implemented and completely verified" might be in the American national interest, they often shift ground and begin charging that even the attempt to negotiate a freeze would be dangerous, because the U.S. might stop building but the Soviets would continue to build. But if the two sides can agree in principle to a freeze, they can also agree to an interim moratorium while the details of the plan are discussed. It would be plain common sense to begin freeze talks with a "negotiator's pause" to hold weaponry constant. A similar pause was put in place and it was effective prior to the 1963 test-ban negotiations.

And sometimes critics even suggest that a nuclear weapons freeze will not, by itself, eliminate the danger of nuclear war. The freeze which they first assailed as too ambitious is then attacked as insufficient to be meaningful. In reality, it is a first but essential step back from the nuclear precipice; it can stop the arms race from rushing over the edge of that precipice, and subsequent reductions can truly move us back to a safer place, farther from the brink.

When these arguments do not avail, the opponents of a freeze offer a counterfeit version, such as the Jackson–Warner resolution introduced in the Senate this spring and supported by the Reagan administration, which calls for a freeze at "equal" levels after "sharp" reductions in nuclear arsenals. This is a false freeze which begins with the assertion that there is, at present, "a nuclear force imbalance." The implication is that the United States must build more to catch up and only then negotiate reductions, or that the Soviets must agree to "unequal reductions," in the phrase of administration arms negotiator Eugene Rostow. According to that scheme, the Soviet Union would give up more of its strategic power than the United States. The prospect for such a negotiating posture hardly seems bright. In any case, lengthy negotiations for reductions before a freeze could lead to frantic production and development of new weapons in the meantime, as each side seeks bargaining chips and marginal advantages. A false freeze calls for running faster before we stop. It is a recipe for putting off the freeze and getting on with the arms race.

Freeze opponents who offer these counterfeit resolutions concede a critical point. By favoring a freeze later, they have, in effect, admitted that a freeze as such is feasible and verifiable. They have agreed to the principle; now they are only haggling about the timing. But ordinary citizens increasingly understand how vital an issue timing is. They are not interested in a "freeze" that is only a cover for another round of the arms buildup; they want a real freeze, and they want it *as soon as possible, as comprehensive as possible*. The Kennedy-Hatfield resolution may not prevail immediately in the Congress or inside the administration, but the people can, and will, keep the pressure on. They will organize, raise their voices, and cast their votes.

The Kennedy-Hatfield resolution, by combining a mutual freeze and major reductions, provides the most promising way to move back the hands of the Doomsday Clock. It is time, perhaps the last period of time we shall have, to cease debating the preferred options of certain experts and public figures who think that there is a better way to dot the *i*'s or cross the *t*'s of arms control. The freeze concept has the inestimable political virtues of simplicity and practicality. Its benefits to humanity are readily apparent to ordinary human beings, rather than to only a select handful of scientists and strategic analysts. There would be no mistaking the moral implications of an agreement to stop the arms race now, and an intense national and international campaign for ratification could be effectively mounted. To a world increasingly apprehensive over the awesome dangers and technological complexities of the arms race, a freeze offers the symbol and the substance of hope.

9

50 QUESTIONS AND ANSWERS ON THE NUCLEAR FREEZE

"You see things and you say 'Why?' But I dream things that never were and I say 'Why not?' "

—George Bernard Shaw

In debates across the country, many have seen the risk of nuclear war and said: "Why?" They've thought about the nuclear freeze and said: "Why not?" Asking and answering such questions is an important part of involvement in the freeze movement. Every concerned citizen can and should have the answers. We hope that these 50 questions and answers will prove to be a good beginning, but to further support your arguments you need only to refer back to the appropriate chapters.

QUESTION 1: How serious is the risk of nuclear war?

ANSWER: More serious today than ever before. Nuclear competition has sometimes led to crisis, as happened after the Soviet installation of missles in Cuba in 1962. From such confrontations war can always erupt, even if it is not desired by either side. Post-World War II technology has reduced the warning time of a nuclear attack from ten hours (for bombers) to ten minutes (for European theater missiles and sub-

144

marine-based missiles); these developments have increased prospects of a nuclear first strike or an accidental nuclear war, while decreasing prospects for halting a nonnuclear conflict before it escalates into a nuclear one. Most serious of all is the danger that one side may suddenly be gripped by a "use them or lose them" psychology in a crisis, fearing that its missiles are about to be destroyed by the other side in a nuclear high noon.

QUESTION 2: Can a nuclear weapons freeze really make a difference in preventing nuclear war?

ANSWER: The freeze is not a cure-all. No arms control agreement can eliminate all risk of nuclear war, but a freeze can stop the present situation from getting worse. A comprehensive freeze would halt the development of new weapons and preclude the acquisition of a dangerous first-strike capability by either side. Citizens will have to make an informed judgment as to whether, all things being equal, they are safer with a continuing arms race or with a halt to the arms race. We think the answer is obvious.

QUESTION 3: Would the freeze perpetuate an unfair or dangerous balance of power?

ANSWER: The freeze would not be unfair to either side, because both the United States and the Soviet Union are effectively equivalent in strategic nuclear power. Each has far more than enough power to retaliate against the other in any possible circumstance. We are ahead in some areas, and they are ahead in others. But the present strategic balance gives us the best opportunity we may ever have to call a halt to in the nuclear arms race. The United States has 9400 strategic nuclear warheads and the Soviet Union has 7500. Even if the Soviets struck first, and their attack worked perfectly, at least 4000 American nuclear warheads in submarines and on bombers would survive—more than enough to turn the Soviet Union into a nuclear wasteland.

QUESTION 4: But shouldn't we wait to freeze the arms race until we catch up to the Russians in areas where we are now behind?

ANSWER: We just answered that. That is the argument of the Reagan administration and of antinuclear freeze proposals like the Jackson-Warner resolution. It simply won't work. One side or the other will always want to build more missiles. Neither will stand still while the other keeps building. Both sides have different types of strategic forces; the Soviets have a greater proportion of land-based missiles, but such missiles are potentially vulnerable; the U.S. relies more on submarine-based missiles, which are more survivable. Overall, however, the two sides are at rough parity, so a freeze can and will work.

QUESTION 5: Shouldn't we at least strive for reductions in Soviet ICBM megatonnage before trying to end the arms race in general?

ANSWER: The U.S. has more strategic nuclear warheads— almost 2000 more, in fact—and warheads are the measure that counts the most. The Soviets have larger missiles that can lift bigger warheads: they have more "throw-weight." But that is partly a result of our greater technical skill, which has enabled us to build smaller, more efficient missiles and warheads. The difference in throw-weight is also largely irrelevant to the real strategic balance, since the accuracy of American missiles means that our firepower does not depend on a larger blast, farther away from the target. In recent years the Defense Department itself has chosen to rely more heavily on smaller and more accurate warheads.

QUESTION 6: Some critics have suggested that a freeze is a bad idea because it will stop us from building new weapons like the M-X, which provide a real incentive for the Soviets to agree to arms reductions. Are they right?

ANSWER: This is "voodoo arms control," which says you must have more in order to have less. It is the old bargaining chip dodge. For example, the last refuge of the pro-ABM lobby before the ABM Treaty was signed was "Give us ABM as a bargaining chip now so that we can negotiate it away later in talks with the Soviet Union." We don't have to build more weapons and make the Russians feel more vulnerable, in order to induce them to enter serious negotiations. If we are perpared to dismantle some of our threatening nuclear weapons, of which we already have thousands, we have all the bargaining chips we need to bring the Russians to the bargaining table. In fact, a U.S. buildup is more likely to drive the Soviets into building more weapons than it is to co-erce them into bargaining. Their buildups have the same effect on us. When more weapons can be rationalized as a way of having fewer weapons, when the word "freeze" can be manipulated to mean an arms race now and a halt postponed to the indefinite future, we have turned rationality upside down and come very close to George Orwell's prophecy for 1984.

QUESTION 7: Without a freeze, will the balance of nuclear power shift toward us or away from us?

ANSWER: There is no guarantee that the U.S. wlil be in a better position in the arms race tomorrow than it is today. Both sides have drifted into *worse* positions while the arms race rushes ahead. In effect, *both* sides are behind! If nuclear war broke out now, the U.S. and the Soviet Union would suffer more destruction than they would have 10 years ago, and far, far more than 20 years ago. At this stage of the arms race, the U.S. is straining its resources to develop and deploy the M-X, to build a new strategic bomber, and to modernize its missile-firing submarines. The Soviets have been engaged in their own large buildup, and there is no reason to think they will stand still while we keep building. We will be worse off, even in relative terms, if we wait another decade before proposing a freeze.

QUESTION 8: Won't a nuclear weapons freeze give the Soviet Union an advantage, since they have more conventional forces?

ANSWER: A freeze won't stop the Red Army, or start it. In terms of the power balance, it will leave both sides where they are today. We will still have a powerful nuclear deterrent, but more resources will be available to strengthen our conventional forces.

QUESTION 9: How much money will a freeze save?

ANSWER: Our spending on nuclear weapons averages about $35 billion a year. About half of that amount will be saved by a freeze: $18 billion a year, or $90 billion over the next five years. If negotiated reductions follow, there will be substantial additional savings in the cost of operating and maintaining nuclear weapons. Some of the savings could be applied to our conventional forces; the rest could be used to cut the deficit or to pay for vital social programs.

QUESTION 10: Do enough people support a freeze to make it possible?

ANSWER: Yes. The freeze movement has struck a deeply responsive public chord. The Reagan administration is digging in its heels. The people are ahead of the politicians, but you can make them catch up. You have a voice and a vote. The outcome is up to you.

QUESTION 11: Has a nuclear weapons freeze been proposed before?

ANSWER: A freeze was proposed in 1964 by President Lyndon Johnson, when the United States was far ahead in nuclear weaponry. The Russians wouldn't buy it. A freeze was proposed again in a resolution which the Senate passed by a vote of 73 to 6 in 1970, urging President Nixon to seek a freeze on offensive and defensive strategic weapons with the Soviet Union. The Nixon administration rejected the idea.

QUESTION 12: Is there anything in arms control history that suggests a freeze is possible now?

ANSWER: Several treaties already negotiated with the Soviet Union have achieved partial freezes. The Test-Ban Treaty of 1963 froze the testing of nuclear weapons in the atmosphere, in space, or under water; the ABM Treaty of 1972 froze antiballistic missile deployment; and a Comprehensive Test-Ban Treaty, nearly completed before the Reagan Administration suspended the negotiations, would freeze all nuclear testing. In each case, the doubters were proved wrong about the possibility of reaching and ratifying an agreement—and the people helped prove them wrong. Treaties with real popular support were ratified. The 1963 test ban came after years of citizen concern about radioactive fallout from nuclear tests. The ABM Treaty in 1972 came amid public debate about "bombs in the backyard"—an America dotted with antimissile bases. The SALT II Treaty failed in the Senate in 1979 largely because it did not have the broad popular support which the other treaties had.

QUESTION 13: How long can we wait for a freeze?

ANSWER: Waiting won't work. There is no reason to believe that the U.S. can improve its overall strategic position by holding off and building more weapons in the meantime. The Soviets have made it clear that they will not stay on the sidelines while we run another lap in the arms race. They will match any and every American buildup. Neither nation is likely to accept that would be, in effect, a unilateral freeze. Freezing later means bigger arsenals for both sides and greater dangers for us all.

QUESTION 14: If the Reagan administration refuses to propose a freeze, would a freeze still make sense after the 1984 election?

ANSWER: Of course it would; it may take a while to build the necessary support for a freeze in this administration, but if people want it and vote for it in 1982, you may make it happen sooner than you think.

QUESTION 15: Does the Kennedy-Hatfield resolution call for a unilateral freeze?

ANSWER: No. Our resolution calls for a bilateral freeze. But one country has to ask the other to dance. Once there is agreement in principle, both sides can put a moratorium on new weapons while working out the details of verification for a freeze. That kind of "negotiators' pause" was put in place before the 1963 test-ban talks.

QUESTION 16: Should supporters of the SALT II Treaty also support a freeze?

ANSWER: If you liked SALT, you'll love the freeze. A freeze goes well beyond SALT II because it will stop the nuclear buildup now—and not just on some weapons, but on all of them.

QUESTION 17: Why is the Reagan administration opposing a nuclear weapons freeze?

ANSWER: The administration opposes it because of the false notion that America is behind in nuclear weapons. This is plainly wrong; the U.S. has 9400 strategic nuclear warheads and the Soviet Union has 7500—and warheads are the single most important measure of strategic power. No American military leader would trade our strategic forces for those of the Soviet Union. The administration also says that a freeze will perpetuate Soviet nuclear superiority in Europe. In fact, the Kennedy-Hatfield resolution rejects a Europe-only freeze; that would merely invite both sides to divert resources to nuclear buildups in other areas, which has been the pattern of selective agreements for two decades. A comprehensive freeze will stop that deadly pattern. It will not change in any way the NATO doctrine which commits the full strength of the United Stated and the Western Alliance to the defense of Europe.

QUESTION 18: Will a freeze be permanent?

ANSWER: It will set a permanent limit no higher than current levels. But a freeze is only the first step. The second step is negotiated reductions under which each superpower would eliminate its most vulnerable and destabilizing weapons. However, a freeze makes sense by itself. And it would make no sense to end a freeze unilaterally, to retrace that first step and move back toward the nuclear brink.

QUESTION 19: Can we replace weapons under a freeze, or will we be restricted to the ones we already have?

ANSWER: Each side can replace existing weapons on a one-to-one basis. This was the approach under past freeze proposals. Of course, the two sides could agree as well that some weapons, such as particular categories of ICBMs, would not be replaced as they wore out.

QUESTION 20: How will the freeze affect the vulnerability of land-based missiles?

ANSWER: The freeze would prevent certain measures from being taken to repair that vulnerability, but those measures don't really matter anyway. For example, the deployment of antiballistic missiles to defend land-based missiles is costly, destabilizing, ineffective, and destructive of the ABM Treaty. And adding more land-based ICBMs to protect existing ones only invites a bigger Soviet attack.

In fact, the freeze would reduce the vulnerability of land-based missiles by preventing each side from increasing its first-strike threat to the land-based missiles of the other. The only way to improve potential first-strike capability is to test warheads and missiles. A freeze would forbid that.

QUESTION 21: Will the freeze on production prevent any more submarines and bombers from being produced?

ANSWER: The freeze will prohibit any increase in the numbers or power of nuclear weapons. For example, because both sides will almost certainly wish to maintain fleets of missile-firing submarines, at least for the foreseeable future they could replace submarines as they wore out with others of the same type. But neither nation could expand its fleets.

QUESTION 22: Will all testing of nuclear weapons and nuclear weapon delivery systems be prevented by the freeze?

ANSWER: The freeze will ban all testing of new types of nuclear weapons. It will permit only the flight and sea tests needed for maintenance of existing missiles, bombers, and submarines. This is consistent with the basic principle of the freeze: "Stop where you are."

QUESTION 23: Why not try for reductions first, instead of a freeze first?

ANSWER: The effort to negotiate reductions is inherently more complex and difficult. The entire range of weapons systems may have to be reviewed element by element, with each side bargaining for unilateral advantages. The Jackson-Warner antinuclear freeze resolution, for example, calls for a halt to the arms race only at "equal and sharply reduced" levels. But equality is in the eye of the beholder; there is always a tendency for each side to think that it is behind somewhere. Endless debate over equality and how to achieve it means endless negotiations. And during such negotiations, both sides will continue to build, either to acquire bargaining chips or to get a new weapon in under the wire.

Arms control experience has also shown that reduction agreements generally tend to have loopholes that are exploited. Both sides feel compelled to use such loopholes, out of fear that if one nation does not, the other will. Cruise missiles, for example, became an American nuclear priority when the Defense Department realized that they were not barred by the Vladivostok agreement of 1974. Under SALT II, both the M-X and the Trident II missiles could proceed. A freeze is an arms control fail-safe. It will block buildups during negotiations, and it will block any efforts to exploit loopholes after an agreement is reached.

QUESTION 24: How would the reductions following a freeze be carried out?

ANSWER: The Kennedy-Hatfield resolution suggests "annual percentage reductions or equally effective means." Under the percentage method, categories of weapons would be reduced by a fixed amount each year, say 5 to 7 percent. Within a category, the two sides could choose which weapons they wanted to throw away. If each side reduced its arsenal by 7 percent each year, a 50 percent reduction could be achieved in about seven years.

QUESTION 25: How would these reductions help to stabilize the nuclear balance and prevent nuclear war?

ANSWER: The reductions would provide incentives for each side to discard the weapons that are simultaneously most threatening to the other side and most vulnerable to attack. Land-based missiles are the most accurate weapons; but because they are stationary, they are also the easiest target for the enemy to hit. Such missiles are particularly destabilizing because they invite a preemptive strike during a crisis.

QUESTION 26: Will a freeze work without other nations joining in?

ANSWER: Yes, for the foreseeable future. The British and the French have deliverable warheads measured in the hundreds, while the superpowers have 17,000. China has a force so modest that its refusal to participate in past arms control agreements has never deterred the Soviets from doing so.

QUESTION 27: Once a freeze is in place, why would the Soviets agree to reductions? Won't the freeze undermine our "leverage" for reductions?

ANSWER: A mutual freeze is in the interest of both the United States and the Soviet Union. It is not a favor to the Soviets, or a carrot for them. They don't need a freeze *more* than we do. Both sides need it equally, in order to prevent a nuclear war that would destroy both sides equally. The Soviets have economic incentives to agree to a freeze and reductions, because the arms buildup overburdens their economy as much as or more than it does ours. The discredited bargaining-chip theory, which has seldom worked in arms control, should not be used and misused to block a freeze now.

QUESTION 28: What difference will a freeze and reductions make if both sides still have thousands of nuclear warheads left?

ANSWER: Rome wasn't built in a day, but Washington and

Moscow can be vaporized in a moment. A freeze and reductions are the building blocks of peace. It won't happen all at once, but we can stop moving in the wrong direction, and start moving in the right direction. Today the nuclear arms spiral is an important source of tension and danger. Ending that spiral will diminish the probability of nuclear confrontations that could lead to a holocaust. During the freeze and subsequent reductions, attitudes toward what is necessary for deterrence will change. Initially, both superpowers believed that tens, and later hundreds, of nuclear weapons would be enough; only recently did we decide we needed thousands. As the reduction process continues, we will be able to rely on fewer and fewer weapons for deterrence. Meanwhile, every bomb thrown away helps protect the planet.

QUESTION 29: Can a freeze be verified?

ANSWER: Yes. In fact, a freeze can be more verifiable than other arms control agreements. If the two superpowers can add nothing new to their arsenals, then detecting a violation will be easier than if there are complicated rules about the many things they can do. Of course, some aspects of a freeze will be more difficult to verify than others; but the experts who favor a freeze have made a convincing case that so many different parts of the process, such as testing and deployment, can be verified with high confidence that the overall process is capable of catching any significant violation.

QUESTION 30: Will the freeze agreement require on-site inspection and would the Russians agree to it?

ANSWER: Our current intelligence capability is sufficient for independent American monitoring of a freeze on both the testing and deployment of nuclear weapons. For certain aspects of the freeze on production of nuclear weapons, we may want some form of on-site inspection. The Soviet Union has agreed in principle to on-site monitoring and inspection systems in recent negotiations for a Comprehensive Test-Ban Treaty.

QUESTION 31: Even with on-site inspection, could we know where every last bomb in the Soviet Union was?

ANSWER: Of course not. Bombs are relatively small, and some could be hidden. But that would not pose a significant threat; any substantial violation could and would be caught. As former CIA Deputy Director Herbert Scoville explains, "It is hard to see how any clandestine production that would significantly add to these numbers could escape detection by our intelligence."

QUESTION 32: Can major nuclear weapons reductions be verified?

ANSWER: Yes. We already know how to do it. The standing consultative commission created by the first SALT Treaty agreed on ways to monitor the dismantling of existing strategic weapons.

QUESTION 33: Can we trust the Russians to obey a freeze? Haven't they violated other treaties before?

ANSWER: A nuclear weapons freeze will not depend on trust but on independent verification. The freeze and reductions proposed by the Kennedy-Hatfield resolution can be verified by our own intelligence capability. The administration is currently charging the Soviets with violating certain chemical and biological warfare treaties, but in each case, the treaties permit production for research and for defensive purposes, and they do not include the verification requirements developed in the SALT negotiations and the comprehensive test-ban negotiations. The Kennedy-Hatfield resolution calls for such verification requirements.

QUESTION 34: What about "hard" cases for verification, such as cruise missile production and deployment?

ANSWER: At the moment, the U.S. has a long lead in developing modern, small, efficient cruise missiles. Verification is not as challenging for the Soviets as for the U.S., since we have an open society. A freeze now can prevent the Soviets from even beginning to test sophisticated, long-range cruise missiles. Our intelligence analysts have high confidence in a variety of methods to penetrate Soviet secrecy. These methods continue to improve over time, and what may appear difficult to verify now may well become verifiable in the future.

QUESTION 35: Do we have any reason to think that the Soviet Union will agree to a nuclear weapons freeze?

ANSWER: The Soviets agreed to stop atmospheric nuclear

testing in 1963 and they have kept that agreement. They agreed to what amounts to a freeze on antiballistic missile systems, the ABM treaty of 1972, and they have kept that agreement as well. A freeze if in their national security interest, just as it serves our interest.

QUESTION 36: If the Soviet Union is spending so much money on strategic weapons, won't they just continue the arms race and try to run us into the ground?

ANSWER: They can't overtake us technologically or economically. They understand that in any arms race, we have the know-how to match them step for step. At the end of this tunnel, the only light will be a nuclear fireball.

QUESTION 37: Does the impending change of Soviet leadership reduce the prospects for a freeze?

ANSWER: The issue is not only what leaders want, but what circumstances require. The window of opportunity for a freeze agreement is not likely to be closed under new Soviet leadership; the same economic factors that persuaded their predecessors to pursue arms control will still exist. A new leadership also has to face military realities; they will discover that no matter how fast they run in the arms race, they cannot win.

QUESTION 38: Should we link arms control negotiations, including the Kennedy-Hatfield proposals, to Soviet action in Poland and elsewhere?

ANSWER: On this issue, there should be no linkage. We won't enter a nuclear freeze agreement because we like the Soviets or they like us, but because both of us choose existence over extinction. We can respond to Soviet oppression in Poland and elsewhere, and at the same time work to reduce the danger of nuclear war. Both of us supported strong sanctions against the Soviet action in Poland, and then sponsored the nuclear freeze resolution.

QUESTION 39: What if nonnuclear (conventional) defensive weapons are used to undermine the freeze? Would the Soviets be permitted to develop their air defenses to stop our bombers from getting through? Could they modernize their antisubmarine warfare (ASW) in order to hunt down our submarines?

ANSWER: The freeze applies only to nuclear weapons, so it would not specifically cover these defenses. But our deterrent forces are sufficiently strong and diversified in the land, sea, and air legs of the triad that they cannot be defeated by any Soviet defenses in the foreseeable future. In fact, the United States is far ahead of the Soviets in ASW technology, and we are fully capable of matching any of their developments in the future. We can seek agreements barring ASW or air defenses that could destabilize the existing nuclear balance. A precedent for such an agreement is the Anti-ballistic Missile Treaty of 1972, in which the United States and the Soviet Union agreed to limit the development and deployment of these defensive missile systems. A nuclear weapons freeze is not a panacea for all the problems of arms control, but is the essential precondition for halting the nuclear arms race and addressing the issues that remain.

QUESTION 40: What about esoteric weapons, such as lasers and particle beams? Would the freeze stop them?
ANSWER: They are nonnuclear systems and would not be subject to a freeze. But such esoteric weapons are still in early stages of development, and a nuclear freeze would provide incentives for constructive agreements in this area too.

QUESTION 41: Would civil defense be frozen under the freeze?
ANSWER: No, because civil defense is not a nuclear weapon. In any event, the U.S. should abandon the expensive and nonsensical evacuation planning proposed by the Reagan administration. Civil defense has no effect on the strategic balance; it will not permit the U.S. or the Soviet Union to survive a nuclear war.

QUESTION: 42: Are short-range tactical nuclear weapons, intended only for battle field use, covered by the freeze?
ANSWER: All nuclear weapons are covered, strategic as well as tactical, as long as the freeze is mutual and verifiable.

QUESTION 43: Would the freeze affect the proliferation of nuclear weapons to other nations?
ANSWER: Yes, but indirectly. So long as the super powers continue their own nuclear arms race other nations will seek to compete in the race as well. A freeze will make it more

difficult for such nations to justify the acquisition of their own nuclear weapons capability. The United States, the Soviet Union and over 100 other nations have ratified The Non-Profoiliration Treaty (NPT), signed in 1968, under which these nations agree not to transfer or acquire a nuclear weapons capability and to accept international safeguards over their programs for the peaceful use of nuclear energy. Again, a freeze is not a panacea. But it will significantly enhance U.S. and Soviet credibility in pursuing urgently needed steps to obtain greater adherence to the NPT, strengthen international safeguards, restrain reckless commerce in nuclear energy, and enact other anti-proliferation measures.

QUESTION 44: Would the freeze adversely affect the balance of nuclear power in Europe?

ANSWER: Not at all. A freeze limited to Europe would be unacceptable. But a global freeze would not affect the balance, which has rested for many years on the ability of the United States, and its allies to draw on all of their military power, to destroy the Soviet Union in response to any Soviet nuclear attack on Western Europe.

QUESTION 45: Would America gain or lose respect in Europe with a freeze?

ANSWER: We would gain. America's standing in Europe has been undermined by perceptions that the Reagan administration is willing to take nuclear risks and is not serious about arms control. There has been too much loose talk about limited nuclear war and nuclear warning shots. The neutron bomb has also deepened European anxieties. Whether these perceptions are right or wrong, they have clearly taken hold. The very proposal of a nuclear weapons freeze followed by major reductions can help to repair the damage. Today, Europeans are apprehensive that the United States has a weapons policy, but not a peace policy.

QUESTION 46: Shouldn't the public keep its nose out of the experts' business of defense and arms control?

ANSWER: This happens to be a democracy. As we hope you have learned from this book, the issues are understandable. The case for a freeze is compelling. What is at stake is not simply a technical debate, but the very lives of the American people. They have a right to have their say.

QUESTION 47: What is the best short argument for a freeze?

ANSWER: Enough is enough. The United States has ample retaliatory power to defend itself and its allies against any attack. The U.S. and the Soviet are at rough equivalence in nuclear power and already have the capacity to overkill each other many times. This may be our last best chance to stop the nuclear arms race.

QUESTION 48: But if the Russians agree to a freeze, doesn't it have to be a bad idea?

ANSWER: We have negotiated treaties with them before, when it was in their interest as well as ours to reach agreement. Both nations have a vital interest in mutual survival instead of mutual suicide.

QUESTION 49: How can you tell a false freeze from the real thing?

ANSWER: A false freeze calls for a freeze tomorrow, never a freeze today. The Jackson-Warner resolution, for example, talks of a freeze, but permits the nuclear buildup to proceed. The Kennedy-Hatfield resolution, which is supported by the Nuclear Weapons Freeze Campaign, calls for a freeze now.

QUESTION 50: Is there an alternative to a freeze?

ANSWER: Yes, a continued and escalating nuclear arms race, and possibly a nuclear war.

10

WHAT CAN A CITIZEN DO?

"People want peace so much that one of
these days governments had better get out of
their way and let them have it."
—Dwight D. Eisenhower

What can each of you do? The simple answer to that question is—a lot. In fact, if people of all ages continue to organize effectively, they will make the difference between
success and failure of the nuclear freeze movement. Citizens
and communities can develop the case for a freeze in ways
that elected representatives understand very clearly. The possibilities are limitless: they range from public referendums
through local and statewide ballot initiatives to church base-
ment suppers, meetings in senior citizen centers and union
halls, college campus teach-ins, Chamber of Commerce
forums, and door-to-door petitions. Materials that are keyed
to local conditions and concerns can be prepared and distributed. People can be told what a nuclear war will mean to
their own communities. Research foundations, grassroots organizations, and umbrella groups can be formed to coordinate activities. The early effectiveness of the freeze movement
has already demonstrated the ability of committed citizens to
mobilize public opinion for the prevention of nuclear war.
Congressional and national elections can become a referendum, not only on the economy and domestic issues, but on

the issue of individual and national survival in this nuclear age.

The driving force behind the freeze movement is the growing conviction of citizens in every region and every walk of life that a nuclear weapons freeze may be the only real hope for their survival. The breadth of the movement has already demonstrated that the freeze is not the special province of a liberal or conservative philosophy. The Kennedy-Hatfield nuclear freeze resolution in Congress has drawn support from both parties and across the philosophical spectrum. In no sense is the freeze a special interest issue; there is nothing in it for those who join the effort except the most important thing of all, survival for our families, our children, and our country. Even the nuclear arms merchants have been wisely silent about their loss of profits in a freeze. What is happening in community councils across the country as well as in the corridors of Congress is a classic confrontation between the irresistible force of the freeze idea and the immovable object of the nuclear status quo. Among those who support that status quo are many from the professional elites who have guided America's nuclear strategy for four decades since Hiroshima. They prefer to manage the arms race, rather than end it. In fact, they may be ending western civilization.

As we write this chapter, the freeze movement is entering a critical second stage. The experts have noticed it; some have rallied to it and others have opposed it. Alternative resolutions have been offered in Congress in an attempt to kill the freeze by subverting it from within. Some people want to "build now, freeze later" on the false premise that we need more and bigger and better missiles to catch up with the Soviet Union. Others want to "freeze this, not that," on the foolish premise that the Soviets will agree to a freeze in areas where they are behind, even though the United States keeps building new nuclear weapons in areas where our experts claim we are behind. They want their MX missile, B-1 bomber, and Trident II submarine, but they want the Soviets to stand still.

The nuclear freeze movement is a rarity in twentieth-century America in two respects: its pure spontaneity and its power as a public phenomenon. As such, it is comparable in American history to our movement for independence in the eighteenth century that gave birth to the nation; to the movement to abolish slavery in the nineteenth century that saved the nation; and to the movements in recent years for civil rights, the equal rights of women, and an end to the Vietnam war. The freeze campaign is the ultimate environmental movement. All of these past popular movements raised fundamental questions that could be resolved only by a fundamental break with the status quo. The issue of the nuclear age is perhaps the most fundamental of any age, and citizens have come to understand two things: nuclear war offers no resolution of conflict, but annihilation; and on this issue, people are divided only from their leaders, not among themselves.

If you want to become involved in the freeze movement, there are things that not only need to be done, but that can be tailored to your abilities, your schedule, and your community. The first thing to remember is that you are not alone and you do not have to reinvent the wheel. Some things that can help will occur naturally; others involve the same sort of day-to-day activities that generate public support on any issue, let alone on this most important issue of all. Still other things can be done with a little guidance from organized groups already operating in your area or from the national groups that have been created as a central resource to service you and other involved citizens. As a primer, here are a dozen suggestions that can get you started.

One, know your stuff about the freeze. When your neighbor or your jogging partner wonders whether a freeze will play into the hands of the Russians, be ready to reply that a freeze can work, because the United States is ahead in some areas and the Soviets are ahead in others, but both countries are equal overall. There is only one true freeze; it calls for a mutual freeze *now* with the Soviet Union. Beware of any false freeze that would simply perpetuate the nuclear arms race in disguise.

Two, contact the nearest nuclear freeze chapter and ask what you can do in your area. Volunteer activities range from door-to-door canvassing, telephone polling, and licking envelopes to organizing discussions and providing speakers for groups that request it. If there is no local freeze chapter in your area, consider starting up one of your own. You can find out how by contacting the national or state office of the National Freeze Campaign. The National Freeze Clearinghouse is in St. Louis, Missouri. A complete list of names, addresses, and some telephone numbers of all the chapters in the movement, and of other organizations which are working for nuclear arms control can be found in Appendix C. All of these organizations will help you work for a nuclear freeze. They can offer information, advice, and expertise. With their assistance, you can do the other things that need to be done.

Three, as you begin to get involved, test your ideas and the interest of your friends by hosting a small coffee session in your home or your apartment on the issue. Ask one of the guests ahead of time to make a brief presentation and ask another to lead the discussion.

Four, organize a specific event in your town or high school to educate the public about the freeze. You will be surprised at the amount and quality of help available. In November 1981, the Union of Concerned Scientists sponsored teach-ins on campuses across the country, offered organizational suggestions, and provided a list of speakers, a slide show, and information leaflets. Physicians for Social Responsibility has produced a half-hour film called "The Last Epidemic" for general distribution, describing the effect of a nuclear explosion on San Francisco. 12,000 members belong to the organization, and one in your area will join you to discuss the film. You can also organize local petition drives and conduct freeze workshops to advise others of the actions they can take. Send the signed petitions to your city councils, your state legislators, and the Congress.

For example, a petition to state or local officials might read: We, the undersigned, urge you to support an immediate and comprehensive, mutual, and verifiable nuclear weapons freeze between the United States and the Soviet Union. A petition to a member of Congress might simply read: Please support the Kennedy-Hatfield nuclear freeze resolution.

Five, if you cannot help with time, help with a financial contribution. It takes substantial effort to spread the word, and that effort cannot be made on a shoestring. If you do not know where to send a contribution, mail your check to one of us at 418 C Street, N.E., Washington, D.C., 20002, and we will be sure it gets to a nuclear freeze organization.

Six, involve family, friends, co-workers, and others too. Don't wait for them to raise the issue first. The freeze has already come a great distance by word of mouth, and it will continue to travel this way. It turns out that people care very deeply about preventing nuclear war; in fact, as someone remarked to us, "If you don't care about this issue, you may already be dead!" More than with any other current issue, people are ready to join in on an initiative and work to make it succeed.

Seven, write a letter supporting the freeze to the editor of your daily or weekly newspaper. Comment on a news article, an editorial or an opinion column on the subject, or write out of the blue; you don't have to wait for a development on the issue to occur; just put your views on paper and mail them in. The most eloquent testimonies at Senate hearings are from ordinary citizens who know what they think and who speak from their hearts.

Eight, invite local newspapers and radio and television stations to cover any public event you plan in connection with the freeze. They will often be interested, and they may not always know in advance that you are doing something special. Just call the assignment editor at the paper or news directors at your local stations. Tell them the time and place of the event and inform them of any speakers who are scheduled or any vote that is planned.

Nine, let President Reagan know that you support the Kennedy-Hatfield nuclear weapons freeze proposal, and ask the President to make the freeze the official policy of the United States Government. All you have to do is drop a postcard or a letter in the mail to him in Washington. The address is: President Ronald Reagan, The White House, Washington, D.C. 20500. If you can afford the higher cost, you can send a telegram or a mailgram to the President. You can even place a telephone call directly to the White House. Save money by dialing the telephone number yourself: (202) 456-1414. The cost of a long-distance telephone call from Los Angeles to the White House in the daytime on a weekday is about seventy-five cents for the first minute and about fifty cents a minute after that; the cost is much lower after five o'clock in the afternoon and on weekends. You may never spend a wiser dollar.

Of course you won't get through to President Reagan on the telephone, but the White House switchboard will receive your call and you can leave a specific message about the freeze. The President's staff keeps an accurate record of all the calls, mail, and other communications the White House receives on every issue; they will certainly know you made the effort to reach the President about the freeze.

Ten, let each of your Senators and Representatives in Congress know that you support the freeze. The Kennedy-Hatfield Resolution now has over 190 sponsors in the United States Senate and House of Representatives, primarily because they have heard the message from people like you. Members of Congress think more carefully about issues when they think that your vote in the next election will depend on how they answer you today. You have two Senators representing you and your entire state in the Senate, and one person, chosen in the congressional district in which you live, representing you and your district in the House of Representatives. In all, there are 100 Senators and 435 Representatives, with the number from your state determined by its population. Members of the House of Representatives are elected for two-year terms and Senators are elected for six-year terms, so there will be elections in November 1982 to fill all 435 seats in the House of Representatives but only 33 of the 100 seats in the Senate. Here is the list of the 33 states in which Senate elections will be held in November 1982:

Arizona	New Mexico
California	New Jersey
Connecticut	New York
Delaware	North Dakota
Florida	Ohio
Hawaii	Pennsylvania
Indiana	Rhode Island
Maine	Tennessee
Maryland	Texas
Massachusetts	Utah
Michigan	Virginia
Minnesota	Vermont
Mississippi	Washington
Missouri	West Virginia
Montana	Wisconsin
Nebraska	Wyoming
Nevada	

There are several ways to let your Senators and Representative know how you feel about the nuclear weapons freeze: you can send a postcard, letter, or mailgram to their offices; you can place a telephone call to them; you can even ask them to meet formally or informally with you or your local freeze group. You can contact them in your Washington office, or in their office in your state or in your congressional district. You can call or write or meet with them more than once as developments occur.

When you write, you don't have to say much. A sentence on a postcard—"Please support the Kennedy-Hatfield nuclear weapons freeze"—is enough to get the message through, but the more you say, the more it helps. If you hear on the TV news or read in the newspaper that your Senators or Representatives are against the freeze, call their local office and register your disagreement. Make them realize you feel strongly about the freeze and that it is not just a minor issue, but one of the most important issues of all. Try to talk to them directly by phone or personally in their offices; but if you can't reach them, don't give up without leaving a specific message asking them to support the freeze. Usually, there will be a staff assistant who knows about the freeze and who can talk to you. You can be sure that your Senators and your Representative will be keeping an accurate record of how their constituents feel about the nuclear freeze resolution. It already has their attention, and it won't take a two-by-four to make them notice you.

Ask them specifically to support the Kennedy-Hatfield nuclear freeze resolution. You can also cite the resolution by its number in Congress: Senate Joint Resolution 163 in the United States Senate, and House Joint Resolution 434 in the House of Representatives. Don't just ask them to vote for it; ask them to add their names as actual sponsors of the freeze resolution if they have not already done so. Since 190 members of Congress are now sponsors, your Senators and Representatives will have plenty of company. If you find that they are already sponsoring the resolution, thank them and then politely urge them to work for its passage and enactment into law. If you care about a true freeze, be careful when Senators and Representatives tell you they support the concept of a freeze but prefer a resolution other than the Kennedy-Hatfield resolution; the chances are that they are referring to one of the false freeze resolutions introduced in Congress that will delay the freeze while more and bigger nuclear weapons are produced. Remind them that you want a freeze *now*, which is what the Kennedy-Hatfield resolution calls for. Remember, those who represent you in Congress often oil the wheel that squeaks the loudest; even if you have trouble getting your message across, don't give up or give in.

On this issue, perhaps more than any other, the more they hear from you, the more responsive they will be.

The only address you need to write your Senators in Washington is: His or Her Name, United States Senate, Washington, D.C. 20510. For members of the House of Representatives, write to them in Washington at this address: His or Her name, House of Representatives, Washington, D.C. 20515. You can find a list of every senator and representative in Appendix D.

Remember when you write or call your Senators and your Representative: *you vote, and they have to listen to you.* The day the Congress passes the Kennedy-Hatfield nuclear freeze resolution will be the day the administration decides that it has to pay attention too.

Eleven, lobby your state and local officials and private organizations about the freeze, and ask them to give their official endorsement. It isn't enough to tell your Senators and your Representative in Congress. You can also write and talk with members of your state legislature, your mayor, city councilor, alderman, and others elected to serve you. Don't just tell them how you feel about the freeze; ask them to do something about it, such as signing their names as cosponsors of freeze resolutions in their legislative bodies, or introducing a bill or resolution of their own.

Find out the procedure you need to use and try to get the issue of the freeze on the agenda for the next town meeting or city council session in your area. Go a step further and try to get a referendum for the freeze on the ballot at the next local or state election, just as the freeze supporters in California have. Terry Browne of Lincoln, Massachusetts, described the successful effort by a newly formed freeze group in his community to put the issue on the agenda for their town meeting. He couldn't believe how simple it was: "About thirty members of our three-week-old Lincoln Waging Peace Coalition met at a Thursday morning breakfast at the First Parish Church. We had decided to put a nuclear arms moratorium motion on the Lincoln Town Meeting warrant. Someone submitted several possible wordings and we chose one. By nine A.M. Saturday five of us were in front of the supermarket, drugstore, and post office, ready to go. We needed a hundred signatures by Monday. I've had no experience as a political activist and am shy and diffident. I don't even like to ask people for the time. Consequently, I was a little apprehensive and expected to get a lot of Nos. But I didn't. Most people said 'Fine' and some said 'Thank you for doing this.' We'd chosen the most vaguely worded of the alternatives offered us, to be safe, but I found many people were offended because it was too weak. One man said, 'What about nuclear waste. We're creating terrible environmental hazards. Why don't you say something about that?' Another man said, 'Hell no, I won't sign that. I think we need more bombs.' Some avoided my eyes and hurried to their car. I didn't ask them. And if people said no, I didn't ask why but rapidly turned my attention elsewhere. But five out of six were glad to sign." Hundreds of other town meetings have already endorsed the freeze in every part of the United States, just as Lincoln did. Your community will probably endorse it too, if someone like you asks your neighbors to go on record.

Follow the same sort of blueprint for action to put the freeze on the agenda at the next meeting of private organizations to which you belong. Ask your local bar association or county medical association or chamber of commerce to endorse the freeze; ask other groups, like local civil rights, union, women's, and environmental groups, to go on record too. The more endorsements the freeze collects, the more likely it is to happen.

Suggestions like these are not really very difficult to carry out. You will probably be surprised, just the way Terry Browne was, at the willingness of most people to support the freeze if you show them something specific they can do. You and your family and your friends can be part of a peaceful chain reaction in your community and throughout the country that will help prevent the chain reaction of a nuclear war.

Twelve, register now for the next election, so that you can vote on election day. Do not make the mistake of voting only in a general election; primaries are important too, sometimes even more important. And make it a point before you vote to know how the candidates feel about the freeze.

The genius of American democracy is that individual citizens can get the attention of their government. As Archimedes said in ancient Greece, the birthplace of democracy, "Give me a lever and a place to stand, and I will move the world." The nuclear freeze movement is the lever to move the world away from nuclear destruction. And every American in every corner of America has a place to stand, right in his own community. No other issue matters more than this.

On every other question, when governments make mistakes, the future can correct them. But if governments make the nuclear mistake, there will be no correction, because there will be no future.

It is up to all of us—the people—to demand that this final, fatal mistake must never be made. Each of us, as individuals and as citizens working together, can stand against the continuing arms race that is hurling us toward nuclear war and stand in favor of a nuclear freeze that can bring us toward peace. Robert Kennedy once wrote, "Each time a man stands up for an ideal, or acts to improve the lot of others, or strikes out against injustice, he sends forth a tiny ripple of hope, and crossing each other from a million different centers of energy and daring, those ripples build a current that can sweep down the mightiest walls of oppression and resistance." Today, men and women across the country have stood up in impressive strength. The nuclear freeze campaign is changing the way America thinks about nuclear war. The ripples of hope from the freeze campaign are building a current that is capable of sweeping down the mighty walls of resistance to nuclear arms control. By their energy and daring, individuals in their own communities have already made an astonishing difference. If they succeed in their campaign, they will make all the difference for all the generations to come.

APPENDIX A

THE KENNEDY-HATFIELD CONGRESSIONAL NUCLEAR FREEZE RESOLUTION AND ITS SUPPORTERS

On March 10, 1982, we introduced the Kennedy-Hatfield resolution (S. J. Res. 163 in the United States Senate and H. J. Res. 434 in the House of Representatives) calling for a nuclear weapons freeze and major reductions in current levels of nuclear weapons. The following is the text of our congressional resolution:

> Whereas the greatest challenge facing the earth is to prevent the occurrence of nuclear war by accident or design;
>
> Whereas the nuclear arms race is dangerously increasing the risk of a holocaust that would be humanity's final war; and
>
> Whereas a freeze followed by reductions in nuclear warheads, missiles, and other delivery systems is needed to halt the nuclear arms race and to reduce the risk of nuclear war;
>
> Resolved by the Senate and the House of Representatives of the United States of America in Congress assembled,
>
> 1. As an immediate strategic arms control objective, the United States and the Soviet Union should:
>
> (a) pursue a complete halt to the nuclear arms race;
>
> (b) decide when and how to achieve a mutual and verifiable freeze on the testing, production, and future deployment of nuclear warheads, missiles, and other delivery systems; and
>
> (c) give special attention to destabilizing

weapons whose deployment would make such a
freeze more difficult to achieve.

   2. Proceeding from this freeze, the United States
and the Soviet Union should pursue major, mutual,
and verifiable reductions in nuclear warheads, missiles, and other delivery systems, through annual
percentages or equally effective means, in a manner
that enhances stability.

As we write this appendix, 24 members of the United
States Senate and 166 members of the House of Representatives have agreed to sign their names as sponsors of the Kennedy-Hatfield resolution. These sponsors are listed state by
state in the following table, so that you can find out whether
your two Senators and your Representative in Congress have
signed up as sponsors. An asterisk before a name means that
the Senator or Representative is also a sponsor of the Jackson-Warner resolution in the Senate or the Carney resolution
in the House, which talk about a freeze but do not want it
yet; as explained in Chapter Seven, these two proposals are
very different from the Kennedy-Hatfield resolution, because
they would let the United States and the Soviet Union continue their nuclear buildups.

THE SPONSORS OF THE KENNEDY-HATFIELD RESOLUTION

Alabama

Alaska

Arizona
Rep. Morris K. Udall

Arkansas
*Sen. Dale Bumpers
Rep. Beryl F. Anthony, Jr.

California
*Sen. Alan Cranston
Rep. Anthony C. Beilenson
Rep. George E. Brown, Jr.
Rep. John Burton
Rep. Phillip Burton
Rep. Tony Coelho

Rep. Ronald V. Dellums
Rep. Julian C. Dixon
Rep. Mervyn M. Dymally
Rep. Don Edwards
Rep. Vic Fazio
Rep. Tom Lantos
Rep. Robert T. Matsui
Rep. Paul N. McCloskey, Jr.
Rep. George Miller
Rep. Norman Y. Mineta
Rep. Leon E. Panetta
Rep. Jerry M. Patterson
Rep. Fortney H. Stark
Rep. Henry A. Waxman

Colorado
Rep. Patricia Schroeder
Rep. Timothy E. Wirth

Connecticut
Sen. Christopher J. Dodd
Sen. Lowell P. Weicker
Rep. Lawrence J. DeNardis
Rep. Samuel Gejdenson
Rep. Barbara Kennelly
Rep. Stewart B. McKinney
Rep. Toby Moffett
Rep. William R. Ratchford

Delaware

Florida
Rep. Dante B. Fascell
Rep. William Lehman
Rep. Claude D. Pepper

Georgia
Rep. Wyche Fowler, Jr.

Hawaii
*Sen. Daniel K. Inouye
Sen. Spark M. Matsunaga
Rep. Daniel K. Akaka

Idaho

Illinois
Rep. John G. Fary
*Rep. Lynn M. Martin
Rep. Marty Russo
Rep. Gus Savage
Rep. Paul Simon
Rep. Harold Washington
Rep. Sidney R. Yates

Indiana
Rep. Adam Benjamin, Jr.
Rep. David W. Evans
Rep. Lee H. Hamilton
*Rep. Andrew Jacobs, Jr.

Iowa
Rep. Berkley Bedell
Rep. Cooper Evans
Rep. Tom Harkin
Rep. Jim Leach
Rep. Neal Smith
Rep. Thomas J. Tauke

Kansas
Rep. Dan Glickman

Kentucky
Sen. Walter (Dee) Huddleston
Rep. Romano L. Mazzoli

Louisiana
Rep. Gillis W. Long

Maine
Sen. George J. Mitchell

Maryland
Sen. Paul S. Sarbanes
Rep. Michael D. Barnes
Rep. Steny H. Hoyer
Rep. Barbara A. Mikulski
Rep. Parren J. Mitchell

Massachusetts
Sen. Edward M. Kennedy
Sen. Paul E. Tsongas
Rep. Edward P. Boland
Rep. Silvio O. Conte
Rep. Brian J. Donnelly
Rep. Joseph D. Early
Rep. Barney Frank
Rep. Margaret M. Heckler
Rep. Edward J. Markey
Rep. Nicholas Mavroules
Rep. John Joseph Moakley
Rep. James M. Shannon
Rep. Gerry E. Studds

Michigan
Sen. Carl Levin
Sen. Donald W. Riegle, Jr.
Rep. Daniel J. Albosta
Rep. James J. Blanchard
Rep. David E. Bonior
Rep. William M. Brodhead
Rep. John Conyers, Jr.
Rep. George W. Crockett, Jr.
Rep. William D. Ford
Rep. Dale E. Kildee
Rep. Bob Traxler
Rep. Howard E. Wolpe

Minnesota
Rep. James L. Oberstar
Rep. Martin O. Sabo
Rep. Bruce F. Vento

172 FREEZE!

Mississippi

Missouri
Sen. Thomas F. Eagleton
Rep. Richard Bolling
Rep. William (Bill) Clay

Montana
Sen. Max Baucus
*Sen. John Melcher
Rep. Pat Williams

Nebraska

Nevada

New Hampshire
Rep. Norman E. D'Amours

New Jersey
Rep. Bernard J. Dwyer
Rep. Millicent Fenwick
Rep. James J. Florio
*Rep. Edwin B. Forsythe
Rep. Frank J. Guarini
Rep. Harold C. Hollenbeck
Rep. James J. Howard
Rep. William J. Hughes
Rep. Joseph G. Minish
Rep. Peter W. Rodino, Jr.
Rep. Robert A. Roe
Rep. Christopher H. Smith

New Mexico
Rep. Manuel Lujan

New York
*Sen. Daniel Patrick Moynihan
Rep. Joseph P. Addabbo
Rep. Mario Biaggi
Rep. Jonathan B. Bingham
Rep. Shirley Chisholm
Rep. Thomas J. Downey
Rep. Geraldine Anne Ferraro
Rep. Robert Garcia
Rep. Bill Green
*Rep. Frank Horton
Rep. John J. LaFalce
*Rep. John LeBoutillier
Rep. Stanley N. Lundine
Rep. Matthew F. McHugh
Rep. Henry J. Nowak

Rep. Richard L. Ottinger
Rep. Peter A. Peyser
Rep. Charles B. Rangel
Rep. Frederick W. Richmond
Rep. Benjamin S. Rosenthal
Rep. James H. Scheuer
Rep. Charles E. Schumer
Rep. Stephen J. Solarz
Rep. Ted Weiss

North Carolina
Rep. Ike Andrews
Rep. Walter B. Jones
Rep. Stephen L. Neal

North Dakota
Rep. Byron L. Dorgan

Ohio
Sen. Howard M. Metzenbaum
Rep. Dennis E. Eckart
Rep. Tony P. Hall
Rep. Ronald M. Mottl
Rep. Mary Rose Oakar
Rep. Michael G. Oxley
Rep. Donald J. Pease
Rep. Ralph Regula
Rep. John F. Seiberling
Rep. Bob Shamansky
Rep. Louis Stokes

Oklahoma
Rep. James R. Jones
Rep. Mike Synar

Oregon
Sen. Mark O. Hatfield
Rep. Les AuCoin
Rep. James Weaver
Rep. Ron Wyden

Pennsylvania
Rep. William F. Clinger, Jr.
Rep. James K. Coyne
Rep. William J. Coyne
Rep. Bob Edgar
Rep. Allen E. Ertel
Rep. Thomas M. Foglietta
Rep. William H. Gray III
Rep. Marc L. Marks
*Rep. Austin J. Murphy
Rep. Doug Walgren

Rhode Island
Sen. John H. Chafee
Sen. Claiborne Pell
Rep. Fernand J. St. Germain
Rep. Claudine Schneider

South Carolina

South Dakota
Rep. Thomas A. Daschle

Tennessee
Rep. Harold E. Ford
Rep. Albert A. Gore, Jr.

Texas
Rep. Mickey Leland

Utah

Vermont
Sen. Patrick J. Leahy
Sen. Robert T. Stafford

Virginia

Washington
Rep. Don Bonker

Rep. Norman D. Dicks
Rep. Mike Lowry
Rep. Al Swift

West Virginia
*Sen. Robert C. Byrd
*Rep. Nick J. Rahall II

Wisconsin
Rep. Robert W. Kastenmeier
Rep. Henry S. Reuss

Wyoming

American Samoa

District of Columbia
Delegate Walter E. Fauntroy

Guam

Puerto Rico

Virgin Islands
Delegate Ron de Lugo

DEFENSE, FOREIGN POLICY, AND SCIENTIFIC EXPERTS WHO HAVE ENDORSED THE KENNEDY-HATFIELD NUCLEAR FREEZE RESOLUTION

(Institutional affiliations are listed for identification purposes only)

Dr. Herbert L. Abrams
Chairman, Department of Radiology, Harvard Medical School

Robert Alpern
Chair, Government Relations Task Force, National Nuclear Weapons Freeze Campaign

George Ball
Senior Managing Director, Lehman Brothers, and former Under Secretary of State

174 FREEZE!

Richard Barnett
Senior Fellow, Institute for Policy Studies

Dr. Paul Beeson
Co-Chairman, Physicians for Social Responsibility and Professor of
Medicine, University of Washington

Sandy Berger
Former Deputy Director, Policy Planning Staff, Department of State

Suzanne Berger
Professor of Physics, M.I.T.

Dr. Robert Berliner
Dean, Yale Medical School

Hans Bethe
Nobel Laureate in Physics, former Director, Theoretical Physics Divi-
sion, Los Alamos Scientific Laboratory, and former member,
Presidential Science Advisory Committee

Dr. T. Berry Brazelton
Chief, Child Development Unit, Children's Hospital Medical Center

Harvey Brooks
Professor, John F. Kennedy School of Government Harvard University

Yvonne Brathwaite Burke
Former Member of Congress

Anne H. Cahn, Director
Committee for National Security

Rear Admiral Eugene J. Carroll, U.S.N. (Ret.)
Deputy Director, Center for Defense Information, and former As-
sistant Deputy Chief of Naval Operations for Plans, Policy, and
Operations

Barry E. Carter
Professor, Georgetown Law Center, and former staff member, National
Security Council

Hodding Carter
Former Assistant Secretary of State

Dr. Thomas C. Chalmers
President, Mount Sinai Medical Center and Dean, Mount Sinai School
of Medicine

Abraham Chayes
Professor of Law, Harvard Law School, and former Legal Advisor to
the Department of State

Warren Christopher
Former Deputy Secretary of State and former Deputy Attorney General of the United States

Frank Church
Former Chairman, Senate Committee on Foreign Relations

Harlan Cleveland
Director, Hubert H. Humphrey Institute of Public Affairs, University
    of Minnesota, former Assistant Secretary of State, and former
    Ambassador to NATO

Clark Clifford
Former Secretary of Defense

William Colby
Former Director, Central Intelligence Agency

David Cortwright
Executive Director, SANE

Teana Crassover
Executive Director, Nurses Alliance for the Prevention of Nuclear War

John Culver
Former member, Senate Committee on Armed Services

Rear Admiral Thomas Davies, USN (Ret.)
Former Commander of Carrier Divisions in the Atlantic and Mediter-
    ranean, and Assistant Director, Arms Control and Disarmament
    Agency

Paul Doty
Director, Program on Science and International Affairs John F. Ken-
    nedy School of Government, Harvard University

John Dow
Former Member of Congress

Rear Admiral Henry Eccles, U.S.N. (Ret.)

William Epstein
Consultant to the Secretary General of the United Nations

Major General William Fairbourn, U.S.M.C. (Ret.)
Associate Director, Center for Defense Information, and former Direc-
    tor for Plans and Policy, Joint Chiefs of Staff

Philip Farley
Senior Fellow, Stanford Arms Control and Disarmament Program, and
    former Deputy Director, Arms Control and Disarmament Agency

Bernard T. Feld
Chairman, Executive Committee, Pugwash Conferences Professor of
    Physics, MIT, and Editor, *Bulletin of Atomic Scientists*

George Feldman
Former U.S. Ambassador

Dr. Stuart Finch
Chief, Department of Medicine, Cooper Medical Center, and former
    Director of Research, Radiation Effects Research Foundation

Roger Fisher
Professor of Law, Harvard Law School, and former Consultant to the
    Assistant Secretary of Defense for International Security

Randall Forsberg
Founder, National Nuclear Weapons Freeze Campaign and Director, Institute for Defense and Disarmament Studies, Brookline, Massachusetts

William Foster
Former Director, Arms Control and Disarmament Agency, former Deputy Secretary of Defense, and former Chief U.S. Negotiator, 18-Nation Disarmament Conference

Alton Frye
Senior Fellow, Council on Foreign Relations

J. William Fulbright
Former Chairman, Senate Committee on Foreign Relations

Mark Garrison
Director, Center for Foreign Policy Development, Brown University

General James M. Gavin
Lieut. General U.S. Army (ret.), and former Ambassador to France

Dr. Jack Geiger
Arthur C. Logan Professor of Community Medicine, City College of New York

Marshall Goldman
Associate Director, Russian Research Center, Harvard University, and Professor of Economics, Wellesley College

Dr. David Greer
Director of Community Medicine, Brown University College of Medicine

Jerome Grossman
President, Council for a Liveable World

Morton Halperin
Former Deputy Assistant Secretary of Defense for Policy Planning and Arms Control

W. Averell Harriman
Former Governor of New York, Under Secretary of State, and Ambassador to Great Britain and the Soviet Union

Robert Heilbroner
Economist, Professor, New School for Social Research, and former Lecturer, National War College

Dr. Howard Hiatt
Director, Harvard School of Public Health, Harvard University

Stanley Hoffmann
Professor of Government and Chairman, Center for European Studies, Harvard University

Townsend Hoopes
Former Under Secretary of the Air Force, and former Assistant Secretary of Defense for International Security Affairs

Dr. Carl Johnson
Associate Clinical Professor of Preventive Medicine, University of Colorado Medical School

Alan Kay
President, Business Alert to Nuclear War

Edy Kaufman
Department of Political Science, University of California

Randall Kehler
National Coordinator, Nuclear Weapons Freeze Campaign

Henry Kelly
Council Member, Federation of American Scientists

George F. Kennan
Professor Emeritus, Institute for Advanced Studies, Princeton, and former Ambassador to the Soviet Union and Yugoslavia

Kenneth Kenniston
Professor of Science, Technology and Society, MIT

George Kistiakowsky
Professor Emeritus of Chemistry, Harvard University, and former Science Advisor to Presidents Eisenhower, Kennedy, and Johnson

Philip Klutznick
Former Secretary of Commerce

Paul Kreisberg
Director of Studies, Council on Foreign Relations, and former Deputy Director, Policy Planning Staff, Department of State

W. Anthony Lake
Professor of International Relations, Amherst College, and former Director, Policy Planning Staff, Department of State

Rear Admiral Gene R. La Rocque, U.S.N. (Ret.)
Director, Center for Defense Information,—and former Assistant Director, Strategic Plans Division, Office of the Chief of Naval Operations

Dr. Alexander Leaf
Ridley Watts Professor and Chairman of Department of Preventive Medicine, Harvard Medical School

Vice Admiral John M. Lee
Former Assistant Director, Arms Control and Disarmament Agency

Dr. Philip R. Lee
School of Medicine, University of California

Rear Admiral William Lemos, U.S.N. (Ret.)

James F. Leonard
Chairman of the Board, the Committee for National Security and former President, Association for the United Nations, and Deputy Ambassador to the United Nations

Wassily Leontief
Professor of Economics, New York University, and Nobel laureate

John W. Lewis
Professor of Political Science, and Director, Arms Control and Disarmament Program, Stanford University.

Robert Lieber
Professor of Government, Georgetown University

Robert J. Lifton
Professor of Psychiatry, Yale University

David Linebaugh
Former Deputy Assistant Director, Arms Control and Disarmament Agency

Sol Linowitz
Former Ambassador to the Organization of American States and Special Envoy to the Middle East

Henry Cabot Lodge
Former Ambassador to the United Nations and Germany, and former Head of the United States Delegation to the Vietnam peace talks

Amory Lovins
Author, Visiting Professor, Dartmouth College, and energy consultant, Friends of the Earth

Dr. Bernard Lown
Professor of Cardiology, Harvard School of Public Health and Co-President, International Physicians for the Prevention of Nuclear War

Patrick J. Lucey
Former Ambassador

Dr. John E. Mack
Professor of Psychiatry, Harvard Medical School

Carl Marcy
Co-Director, American Committee on East-West Accord and former Staff Director, Senate Foreign Relations Committee

Dr. Judd Marmor
Professor Emeritus of Psychiatry, University of Southern California School of Medicine

Jeanne B. Mattison
Co-Director, American Committee on East-West Accord

Former Senator George McGovern
Chairman, Americans for Common Sense

Donald McHenry
Professor, School of Foreign Service, Georgetown University, and former Ambassador to the United Nations

Thomas McIntyre
Former Member, Senate Committee on Armed Services

Leonard Meeker
Member, Board of Directors, Union of Concerned Scientists, and former Legal Advisor, Department of State

Seymour Melman
Professor of Economics, Columbia University

Dr. Karl Menninger
Menninger Foundation and Villages, Inc.

Matthew Meselson
Professor of Biochemistry and Molecular Biology, Harvard University

Elliot L. Meyrowitz
Executive Director, Lawyers Committee on Nuclear Policy

Philip Morrison
Professor of Physics, MIT

Dr. David Nathan
Children's Hospital Medical Center

Former Senator Gaylord Nelson
Chairman, Wilderness Society

Edward Purcell
Professor of Physics, Harvard University, and Nobel laureate in physics

Marcus Raskin
Co-Director, Institute for Policy Studies

George Rathjens
Professor of Political Science, MIT and former Director of Weapons Systems Evaluation Division, Institute for Defense Analysis

Carl Sagan
Astronomer, Cornell University

Harrison Salisbury
Soviet scholar and former diplomatic correspondent, *New York Times*

Dr. Jonas Salk
Founding Director and Resident Fellow, Salk University for Biological Studies

John C. Sawhill
Director, McKinsey and Co., former President, New York University, and Deputy Secretary of Energy

Robert D. Schmidt
President, American Committee on East-West Accord

Herbert Scoville, Jr.
Former Deputy Director for Research (Science and Technology), Central Intelligence Agency, and Assistant Director, Arms Control and Disarmament Agency

Jane Sharp
Professor, Peace Studies Program, Cornell University

Stanely K. Sheinbaum
Economist and Chairman, ACLU of Southern California

Alan B. Sherr
President, Lawyers Alliance for Nuclear Arms Control

Marshall Shulman
Director, Russian Research Institute, Columbia University, and former Senior Advisor to the Secretary of State

Dr. Victor Sidel
Professor and Chairperson, Department of Social Medicine, Montefiore Hospital and Medical Center

J. David Singer
Professor of Political Science, University of Michigan

Eugene Skolnikoff
Chairman of the Board, German Marshall Fund, and Director, Center of International Studies, MIT

Gerard Smith
Former Director, Arms Control and Disarmament Agency, and Chief SALT negotiator

Dr. Leonard Solon
Director, Bureau for Radiation Control, New York City Department of Health

Gus Speth
Georgetown Law Center; former Chairman, U.S. Council on Environmental Quality

John Steinbruner
Director of Foreign Policy Studies, Brookings Institution

Jeremy J. Stone
Director, Federation of American Scientists

Alice Tepper-Marlin
Council on Economic Priorities

Dr. Lewis Thomas
Chancellor, Memorial Sloan-Kettering Cancer Center

Stephen Thomas
Integrative Biomedical Research

Lester Thurow
Professor of Economics, MIT

Richard Ullman
Professor of International Relations, Woodrow Wilson School, Princeton University, and former Editor, *Foreign Policy* Magazine.

George Wald
Nobel laureate, and Professor of Biology, Harvard University

Paul Warnke
Former Director, Arms Control and Disarmament Agency, Chief SALT negotiator, and Assistant Secretary of Defense

Thomas J. Watson Jr.
Former Chairman of the Board, IBM, Ambassador to the Soviet Union,

and Chairman of the General Advisory Committee, Arms Control and Disarmament Agency

William Wickersham
Executive Director, World Federalists Association

Jerome B. Wiesner
Past President, MIT, and Science Advisor to President Kennedy

Christopher Wright
Carnegie Institution of Washington

Adam Yarmolinsky
Former Counselor to the Arms Control and Disarmament Agency, and former Special Assistant to the Secretary of Defense

Herbert F. York
Professor of Physics, University of California, former Negotiator for the Comprehensive Test-Ban Treaty, Director of Defense Research and Engineering, and Director of Lawrence Radiation Laboratory

Andrew Young
Mayor of Atlanta, and former Ambassador to the United Nations

RELIGIOUS LEADERS AND RELIGIOUS ORGANIZATIONS WHICH HAVE ENDORSED THE KENNEDY-HATFIELD NUCLEAR FREEZE RESOLUTION

(Institutional affiliations of individuals are listed for identification purposes only)

Dr. Thelma Adaire
President, Church Women United

Jimmy R. Allen
Former President, Southern Baptist Convention

Father Thomas Ambrogi
Director of Social Justice
Archdiocese of San Francisco

American Friends Service Committee

Zelle Andrews
Peace Advocacy Project Director
United Church of Christ

Bishop James Armstrong
President, National Council of Churches

Association of American Catholic Colleges and Universities

Baptist Joint Committee on Public Affairs

Helen I. Barnhill
Moderator, United Church of Christ

Bishop George Bashore
United Methodist Church
Boston, MA

Rabbi Leonard Beerman
Co-Chair, Interfaith Center to Reverse the Arms Race

Reverend Asia Bennett
Executive Secretary
American Friends Service Committee

Rabbi Leonard I. Berman
Leo Baeck Temple
Los Angeles, California

Bishop Edwin Boulton
United Methodist Church, Dakotas Area

Rabbi Balfour Brickner
Stephen Wise Free Synagogue
New York, NY

Reverend Arie Brouwer
General Secretary, Reformed Church in America

Dr. Edward Brubaker
Executive for United Presbyterian Church
Synods of Mid-America

Bishop Joseph Brunini
Catholic Diocese of Jackson, MI

Walter H. Capps
Professor of Religious Studies, University of California at Santa Barbara; President, Council on the Study of Religion

Reverend Thomas M. Castlen
Associate Synod Executive
United Presbyterian Church, Cascades Presbytery, OR

Reverend John Chapman
Associate Synod Executive, Synod of the North East
United Presbyterian Church of the U.S.A.

Bishop Otis Charles
Episcopal Diocese of Utah

Clergy and Laity Concerned

Bishop Wayne Clymer
United Methodist Church, IA

Reverend Dr. William K. Cober
Executive Director, Board of Ministries, American Baptist Churches of the U.S.A.

Dr. William Sloan Coffin
Riverside Church, New York, NY

Bishop James R. Crumley, Jr.
President, Lutheran Church of America

Robert E. Cuthill
Synod Executive, Synod of Lakes and Prairies
United Presbyterian Church in the U.S.A.

Ruth Daugherty
President, Woman's Division, United Methodist Church

Reverend Robert Davidson
Moderator, General Assembly
United Presbyterian Church in the U.S.A.

Yvonne Delk
Executive Director
Office for Church in Society
United Church of Christ

Reverend John Dertz
Moderator
Synod of the Piedmont
United Presbyterian Church of the U.S.A.

Bishop Jesse R. De Witt
President, General Board of Global Ministry
United Methodist Church

Dr. James M. Dunn
Executive Director
Baptist Joint Committee on Public Affairs

Gretchen Eick
Policy Advocate
Washington Office
United Church of Christ

Theodore W. Engstrom
Chief Executive Officer
World Vision International

Thom White Wolf Fassett
Associate General Secretary, United Methodist Church

Fellowship of Reconciliation

Bishop Bernard Flanagan
Catholic Diocese of Worcester, MA

Reverend Carl Flemister
Executive Director, American Baptist Association

Friends Committee on National Legislation

Sister Alice Gallen
Executive Director
Association of Catholic Colleges and Universities

Rabbi Joseph Glaser
Executive Vice-President
Central Conference of American Rabbis

Reverend Casper I. Glenn
Synod Executive, United Presbyterian Church in the U.S.A.
Synod of Alaska-Northwest

Rabbi Robert E. Goldburg
Rabbi Emeritus, Congregation Mishkan Israel
New Canaan, CT

Reverend Billy Graham

Bishop Thomas J. Gumbleton,
Catholic Diocese of Detroit, MI

Reverend Richard Halverson
Chaplain, U.S. Senate

Michael Hamilton
Canon, Washington Cathedral

Bishop Timothy Harrington
Catholic Diocese of Worcester, MA

Reverend Timothy S. Healy, S.J.
President, Georgetown University

Reverend Theodore Hesburgh, S.J.
President, University of Notre Dame

Archbishop James Hickey
Catholic Archdiocese of Washington, DC

Bishop Kenneth Hicks
United Methodist Church, AK

Bishop Leroy G. Hodapp
President, Board of Church and Society
United Methodist Church

Bishop William R. Houck
Catholic Diocese of Jackson, MI

Reverend William Howard
Past President, National Council of Churches

Bishop George Hunt
Episcopal Diocese of Rhode Island

Archbishop Raymond Hunthausen
Catholic Archdiocese of Seattle, WA

Archbishop Iakovos, Primate
Greek Orthodox Archdiocese of North and South America

Mary Evelyn Jegen
Executive Director, Pax Christi, U.S.A.

Reverend Carroll D. Jenkins
Synod Executive of the Piedmont
United Presbyterian Church in the U.S.A.

Jesuit Social Ministries

Reverend William A. Jones
President, National Black Pastors Conference

Kenneth Kantzer
Editor, *Christianity Today*

Reverend Richard Killmer
Director, Peacemaking Project
United Presbyterian Church in the U.S.A.

Paul Kittlaus
Director, Washington Office
United Church of Christ

Leadership Conference of Women Religious in the U.S.A.

Jane Leiper
Associate Director
Washington Office
National Council of the Church of Christ in the U.S.A.

Reverend Gasper Lo Biondo
Executive Director, Jesuit School Ministries

Dr. Joseph P. Lowery
President, Southern Christian Leadership Conference

Bishop Roger Mahony
Catholic Diocese of Stockton, CA

Reverend C. J. Malloy, Jr.
General Secretary
Progressive National Baptist Convention, Inc.

Rabbi Bernard Mandelbaum
Executive Vice-President, Synagogue Council America

Reverend Canon Charles Martin
Chairman, Peace Commission
Archdiocese of Washington, DC

Bishop Marjorie S. Matthews
United Methodist Church, WI

Bishop Leroy Matthiesen
Catholic Diocese of Amarillo, TX

Reverend Oscar McCloud
General Director, Program Agency
United Presbyterian Church in the U.S.A.

David E. Morris
Executive Presbyter, Presbytery of Northern Waters
United Presbyterian Church in the U.S.A.

Reverend Margaret Morris
Chairperson, Peacemaking Advisory Committee
United Presbyterian Church in the U.S.A.

Bishop Francis P. Murphy
Catholic Diocese of Baltimore, MD

National Council of Churches

Dr. Robert W. Neff
General Secretary
Church of the Brethren General Board

Jenny A. Noblech
President, Children for Peace

Mary Jane Patterson
Director,
Washington Office
United Presbyterian Church, U.S.A.

Dr. Eugene Pickett
President, Unitarian Universalist Association

Bishop Anthony M. Pilla
Catholic Diocese of Cleveland, OH

Dr. Avery Post
President, United Church of Christ

Presbytery of New York, NY
United Presbyterian Church in the U.S.A.

Reverend David W. Preus
Presiding Bishop, American Lutheran Church

Progressive National Baptist Convention, Inc.

Bishop Francis A. Quinn
Catholic Diocese of Sacramento, CA

Archbishop John Quinn
Catholic Archdiocese of San Francisco

Claire Randall
General Secretary
National Council of Churches of Christ in the U.S.A.

Bishop David Reed
Episcopal Diocese of Louisville, KY

Reformed Church in America

Susan Rhoades
Synod of the Rocky Mountains
United Presbyterian Church in the U.S.A.

Riverside Church Disarmament Program
New York, NY

Reverend Joseph Roberts
Pastor, Ebenezer Baptist Church, Atlanta, GA

Bishop Frank J. Rodimer
Catholic Diocese of Paterson, NJ

Rabbi David Saperstein
Religious Action Center
Union of American Hebrew Congregations

Rabbi Herman Schaalman
President, Central Conference of American Rabbis

Rabbi Alexander M. Schindler
President, Union of American Hebrew Congregations

Reverend Robert Seel
Executive Presbyter, Synod of the Southwest
United Presbyterian Church in the U.S.A.

Reverend John A. Sensenig
Synod of the Rocky Mountains
United Presbyterian Church in the U.S.A.

Ronald Sider
President, Evangelicals for Social Action

Rabbi Henry Siegman
Executive Director, American Jewish Congress

Reverend Simon Smith, S.J.
Jesuit Missions, Inc.

Reverend Robert F. Smylie
Association for Peace and International Affairs
United Presbyterian Church in the U.S.A.

Edward F. Snyder
Executive Secretary
Friends Committee on National Legislation

Sojourners

Bishop Walter F. Sullivan
Catholic Diocese of Richmond, VA

Sister Nancy Sylvester
Legislative Liaison
NETWORK

Synod of the Southwest
United Presbyterian Church in the U.S.A.

William P. Thompson
Stated Clerk, General Assembly
United Presbyterian Church in the U.S.A.

Dr. Daniel Thursz
Executive Vice-President, B'nai B'rith International

Reverend John H. Tietjen
President, Christian Seminary-Seminex

Dr. Eugene Turner
Synod Executive, Synod of the Northeast
United Presbyterian Church in the U.S.A.

United Methodist Church

United Presbyterian Church, General Assembly

Reverend Foy Valentine
Executive Director
Christian Life Commission of the Southern Baptist Convention

Dr. Vernon B. Van Bruggen
Synod of the Northeast
United Presbyterian Church of the U.S.A.

Albert Vorspan
Vice-President, Union of American Hebrew Congregations

Bishop John T. Walker
Episcopal Diocese of Washington, DC

Reverend Paul A. Wee
General Secretary, Lutheran World Ministries

Bishop Frederik Wertz
United Methodist Church, Washington, DC

Reverend Edward A. White
Executive Presbyter
National Capitol Union Presbytery

Reverend Robert White
Minister for Social Issues, Reformed Church in America

Dr. Loretta J. Williams
Unitarian Universalist Association
Boston, MA

Reverend Francis X. Winters, S.J.
Professor of International Relations and of Ethics
Georgetown University

Rabbi Walter S. Wurzburger
President, Synagogue Council of America

Yeates County Area Council of Churches
Social Concerns Committee, Penn Yan, NY

Reverend H. Davis Yeuell
Synod Executive of the Virginias
Presbyterian Church in the U.S.A.

OTHER ORGANIZATIONS WHICH HAVE ENDORSED THE KENNEDY-HATFIELD NUCLEAR FREEZE RESOLUTION

American Association of Colleges for Teacher Education
Suite 610
1 Dupont Circle, N.W.
Washington, DC 20036 (202) 293-2504

American Association of School Administrators
1801 North Moore Street
Arlington, VA 22209 (703) 528-0700

American Public Health Association
1015 15th Street, N.W.
Washington, DC 20005 (202) 789-5600

Business Alert to Nuclear War
Box 7
Belmont, MA 02178 (617) 253-1578

Center for Science in the Public Interest
1755 S Street, N.W.
Washington, DC 20007 (202) 332-9110

Child Welfare League of America
1346 Connecticut Ave., N.W., #310
Washington, DC 20036 (202) 833-2850

Coalition for a New Foreign and Military Policy
120 Maryland Ave., N.E.
Washington, DC 20002 (202) 546-8400

Committee for National Security
1742 N Street, N.W.
Washington, DC 20036 (202) 833-3140

Council for a Livable World
100 Maryland Ave., N.E.
Washington, DC 20036 (202) 534-4100

Critical Mass Energy Project
215 Pennsylvania Ave., S.E.
Washington, DC 20003 (202) 546-4790

Educators for Social Responsibility
Box 7
Brookline, MA 02147 (617) 965-5686

Environmental Action, Inc.
1346 Connecticut Ave., N.W. Rm. 731
Washington, DC 20036 (202) 833-1845

Environmental Policy Center
817 Pennsylvania Ave., S.E.
Washington, DC 20003 (202) 547-5330

Federation of American Scientists
307 Massachusetts Ave., N.E.
Washington, DC 20002 (202) 546-3300

Friends of the Earth
530 7th Street, S.E.
Washington, DC 20003 (202) 543-4312

Greenpeace
2007 R Street, N.W.
Washington, DC 20009 (202) 462-1177

Grey Panthers
3635 Chestnut Street
Philadelphia, PA 19104 (215) 382-3300

High Technology Professionals for Peace
52 Walker Street
Newtonville, MA 02160 (617) 332-9457

Institute for Defense and Disarmament Studies
25 Harvard Street
Brookline, MA 02146 (617) 734-4216

International Physicians for the Prevention of Nuclear War
635 Huntington Ave., Second Floor
Boston, MA 02115 (617) 738-9404

Lawyers Alliance for Nuclear Arms Control
Box 9171
Boston, MA 02114 (617) 727-1036

Lawyers Committee on Nuclear Policy
777 United Nations Plaza, Fifth Floor
New York, NY 10017 (212) 877-8962

League of United Latin American Citizens
400 1st Street, N.W.
Washington, DC 20001 (202) 628-0717

Mexican-American Legal Defense and Education Fund
1411 K Street, N.W.
Washington, DC 20005 (202) 393-5111

National Coalition for Cuban Americans
714 Bonifant Street
Silver Spring, MD 20910 (301) 589-5675

National Committee of the National Nuclear Weapons Freeze
    Campaign
4144 Lindell Blvd.
St. Louis, MO 63801 (314) 533-1169

National Congress of American Indians
202 E Street, N.E.
Washington, DC 20002 (202) 546-1168

National Council of La Raza
1725 I Street, N.W.
Washington, DC 20006 (202) 293-4680

National Tribal Chairman's Association
1010 Vermont Ave., N.W.
Washington, DC 20005 (202) 737-7011

Nurses Alliance for the Prevention of Nuclear War
Box 319
Chestnut Hill, MA 02178 (617) 232-0875

Physicians for Social Responsibility
23 Main Street
Watertown, MA 02172 (617) 924-3468

Pugwash Conferences
305 Massachusetts Ave., N.E.
Washington, DC 20002 (202) 544-1784

SANE
711 G Street, N.W.
Washington, DC 20003 (202) 546-7100

Union of Concerned Scientists
1346 Connecticut Ave., N.W. Suite 1101
Washington, DC 20036 (202) 296-5600

Wilderness Society
1901 Pennsylvania Ave., N.W.
Washington, DC 20006 (202) 828-6600

OTHER INDIVIDUALS WHO HAVE
ENDORSED THE KENNEDY-HATFIELD
NUCLEAR FREEZE RESOLUTION

(Institutional affiliations are listed for identification purposes only)

Ruth Adams
Bulletin of Atomic Scientists

Ed Asner
President, Screen Actors Guild

Joan Baez
President, Humanitas International

Leonard Bernstein
Composer-Conductor

Richard L. Bowditch, Jr.
Business Executive

David Brower
Friends of the Earth

Jack Calhoun
Director for Government Affairs, Child Welfare League of America

Norman Cousins
Author

Ned Crosby
Center for Democratic Processes

James K. Devlin
President and Chairman of the Board, U.S. Telephone Communications, Inc.

Reverend Robert Drinan, S.J.
President, Americans for Democratic Action

Marion Edelman
President, Children's Defense Fund

Russell Edgerton
Executive Director, American Association for Higher Education

Peter Eisenman
Director, Institute for Architecture and Urban Studies

Frances Farenthold
Former President of Wells College

Arnold Fege
Director, Governmental Relations, National Parent-Teachers
    Association

Joseph Filner
Noblemet International

Edwin Firmage
Professor of Law, University of Utah

James L. Fisher
President, Council for Advancement and Support of Education

Robert L. Gale
President, Association of Governing Boards of Universities and Colleges

Galway Ginnell
Poet

C. Gus Grant
Vice-Chairman, Southern Pacific Communications, and President,
    Spacenet

Dr. David Greer
Director of Community Medicine, Brown University College of
    Medicine

Dr. Lester Grinspoon
President, American Psychiatric Association

Antonia Hernandez
Director, Washington Office, Mexican-American Legal Defense and
    Education Fund

Terry Herndon
President, National Education Association

Mildred M. Horton
Former Director, WAVES; Former President, Wellesley College

Alan Houseman
Director, Center for Law and Social Policy

Samuel Husk
Director, Council of Greater City Schools

Dr. David Imig
Executive Director, American Colleges for Teacher Education

John Irving
Novelist

Russell Jim
President, Affiliated Tribes of Northwest Indians

David Jones
U.S. Student Association

Coretta Scott King
President, Martin Luther King Jr. Center for Nonviolent Social Change

Midge Miller
State Representative, Wisconsin

Paul Newman
Actor

Edmund Pellegrino
President, Catholic University

Rafe Pomerance
President, Friends of the Earth

Helen Reddy
Singer

Robert Redford
Actor

Rustum Roy
Materials Research Laboratory, Pennsylvania State University

Eli Sagan
Author

Harvey Seifter
Director, Theater of the New City
New York, NY

Adele Simmons
President, Hampshire College

Ellie Smeal
Chair, National Organization of Women

Roberta Snow
Executive Director, Educators for Social Responsibility

Howard A. Squadron
President, Conference of Major American Jewish Organizations, and
President, American Jewish Congress

Elliot Stein, Jr.
Bastille Properties

Alfred Sunberg
Associate General Secretary, American Association of University
Professors

William Tarlow
Executive, General Mills

A. Stark Taylor, Jr.
Chairman Emeritus, Dallas Cotton Exchange

Jeff Wald
President, The Wald Organization

Stanley Weiss
American Minerals, Inc.

Bernard Weissbourd
Metropolitan Structures

Richard E. Wilson
Vice-President for Governmental Relations, American Association of
Community and Junior Colleges

APPENDIX B

WITNESSES FOR A NUCLEAR FREEZE

The nationwide appeal of the nuclear freeze movement is revealed by the extraordinary grass-roots growth of the freeze campaign and by the eloquent words of distinguished public officials and private citizens who have given their time and their effort to the cause. Members of Congress, religious leaders, leaders of the freeze campaign, and former government and military leaders have spoken with clarity and conviction. They believe that an endless arms race is the wrong answer to the nuclear weapons dilemma, and that the right answer is a nuclear weapons freeze. Here is what they say, as they bear witness for the freeze and for the Kennedy-Hatfield resolution.

Edward J. Markey is a Congressman from Massachusetts who is a principal sponsor of the nuclear freeze resolution in the House of Representatives.

It is clear that members of Congress are hearing from their constituents on this issue. They are telling Congress that the United States and the Soviet Union are on a dangerous nuclear collision course. Both sides have built up gigantic nuclear arsenals. Both sides are developing more and more sophisticated weapons that will be harder and harder to control in a crisis. Both sides are poised to heat up the arms race. It all adds up to one frightening conclusion as far as the public is concerned: We are on the verge of blowing ourselves off the face of the earth. The overkill the superpowers have amassed is mind-boggling. More than 50,000 nuclear warheads are stockpiled on both sides. It would take no more than several hundred of those warheads to effectively destroy life as the United States and the Soviet Union now enjoy it.

And now the U.S. plans to build more nuclear bombs—17,000 more bombs, the largest expansion in warhead production this country has seen in 20 years.

The next generation of U.S. and Soviet nuclear weapons, which will improve each side's ability to knock out the other's missiles in a nuclear exchange, promises to put a hair trigger on nuclear deterrence. In other words, we are developing weapons that could push us into a nuclear war, not keep us out of one.

The arms race between the superpowers also leaves the Americans and Soviets little credibility in persuading other nations to forgo nuclear weapons. As it now stands, more than 30 nations have the capability to build the bomb. Pakistan is preparing to detonate a bomb. Iraq wants the bomb. Libya has a bid to buy the Muslim bomb. By the end of this century, the question we may be asking ourselves is not "Who has the bomb?" but "Who doesn't?"

We're now looking down two paths. The first path is an arms buildup that will have us spending hundreds of billions of dollars on new nuclear weapons. But in the end, all those new nuclear weapons won't buy our children a dime's worth of security. The other path is to sit down with the Soviets and halt this mindless march toward a nuclear holocaust, to sit down and decide how to reduce this awesome capacity of destruction.

Across the country, religious leaders, business executives, lawyers, doctors, college students, and local legislators are organizing to demand a halt to the nuclear arms race. Their message is clear: Enough is enough. The superpowers must reduce their arsenals. We in the Congress must respond to that message. The nuclear weapons freeze resolution calls on the United States and the Soviet Union to negotiate a mutual and verifiable freeze on their nuclear arsenals and then begin major reductions. We must now recognize that the best security for the buck lies at the negotiating table. Building more nuclear weapons merely buys us more trouble. A freeze in the nuclear arms race followed by major reductions is urgently needed—before it is too late.

Silvio O. Conte is a Congressman from Massachusetts and is a principal sponsor of the nuclear freeze resolution in the House of Representatives.

One of the featured excerpts from the life of General Douglas MacArthur shown on NBC's "Sunday Night at the Movies" was the speech he gave regarding the devastating prospects of nuclear war just after the defeat of Japan. He stated then that if we did not take the necessary steps to prevent it, the next major war would lead to Armageddon. Certainly, no one could accuse Douglas MacArthur of fearing a fight or being soft on communism. But he had seen firsthand the awful destruction of Hiroshima and Nagasaki, and he recognized that nuclear warfare would not serve as a viable instrument of national policy. The possibility of worldwide annihilation would become very real. That was nearly 40 years ago. There were only a few bombs then. Now the Soviet Union and the United States possess collectively nearly 17,000 warheads, each vastly more powerful than the Hiroshima-Nagasaki bombs. Only a very small percentage of these 17,000 warheads are required to accomplish the destruction of civilization in the northern hemisphere. The winner of a general nuclear exchange between the Soviet Union and the United States could well be Chile or Brazil, but most certainly not one of the two superpowers. General MacArthur's fears have been realized far behond what he could have imagined.

Coincidentally, CBS's "60 Minutes" on the same Sunday devoted a portion of its broadcast to the testimony of Admiral Hyman Rickover before the Joint Economic Committee in January 1982, upon the eve of his retirement from the Navy. Rickover, the father of our nuclear navy and certainly no dove, stated that he believed that we would, in fact, blow ourselves up in a nuclear war. No matter how you feel about Admiral Rickover's statements—be they self-serving or self-sacrificing—you must grant that he is a one-of-a-kind expert in nuclear arms as well as a dedicated naval officer concerned about our national security. He stated categorically that in analyzing advantages in nuclear weapons as they exist now, numbers do not mean a thing. "What difference does it make whether we have 100 or 200 submarines," he said, "if 100 is enough to do the job." He affirmed over and over again in his testimony that we have enough to do the job of destroying Russia many times over.

The statements of these two seasoned, extremely experienced flag officers are aimed at the heart of our debate today.

Namely, that first, we are headed toward nuclear annihilation; second, the numbers and advantages which accrue to one side or the other simply will not matter in terms of who wins or loses. These are the same conclusions that our constituents are reaching all over the country. It is not just the fringe, or the peaceniks, or the fuzzies, or the "no-nukes" groups that are proposing this freeze. It is the people who support a strong defense, it is the middle ground, it is the solid citizens who are now clearly seeing that the ideas of nuclear superiority or stockpiling or gaining advantage no longer have any meaning in a world where adversaries possess the means to retaliate with surety to any attack. Opponents of the freeze resolution say we must not freeze an advantage in favor of the Russians. I will not answer that argument in terms of nuclear weapons "bean counting." There are many reputable national security proponents who will state that no advantage exists now to either side and that in many areas, the United States still has an edge. Others will violently disagree about who is or is not No. 1. But I will state in the same manner as Admiral Rickover—"So what anyway?" There is no advantage to be gained by making the rubble of an already devastated city bounce higher and higher. There is no addition to our national security from the stockpiling of more and more weapons to the point that the Strategic Air Command staff officer turns to his commander and says, "Sir, we have run out of Soviet targets. What do I do with the rest of these warheads?" I am here to declare to the opponents of a freeze that stockpiling is wasteful silliness which would have some humor attached to it if it were not so dangerous and so expensive.

Still, the opponents will say that if we freeze, then we will not be able to field all of the new nuclear systems that we have coming down the pike that will make the Soviets more vulnerable and give us advantages—such things as the M-X, the B-1, and the Pershing II. My answer is simple. Even if we are behind in some supposed race, a verifiable mutual freeze, which this resolution calls for, will leave us no worse off than we are now. If there are major violations and we cannot stop them, then we can start again from that point. However, if our ultimate aim is the eventual drawdown and elimination of these weapons and if the freeze does work, we will have benefited from not having fielded these new, extremely expensive systems. As long as we maintain the capability to deter the start of a nuclear war with surety, then we can feel safe pursuing and participating in such a freeze. We can do that now and well into the future.

But, you might ask, what about all this recent belief that nuclear war is fightable and winnable. And what about the limited nuclear war. Does not a freeze put us in tremendous jeopardy? As I stated earlier, no general nuclear war is winnable, at least not in the sense of a surviving winner. You can go through the body count and the destruction count if you wish to keep score and declare a winner based on the lowest score. But, I know of no reputable strategist who believes that an effective exchange by both sides will result in what could be truly defined as a victor. Yet, there are those who believe that a limited or special kind of strike is possible that would cause the other side to quit. For instance, many say it is possible to make a limited, surgical strike on our ICBMs, kill only 22 million people and blacken only a small portion of our land. As a result, we would have to surrender because we would risk annihilation if we did not. If we follow that logic, we might as well surrender now and avoid the losses. But that is not now and never has been our national policy. To think otherwise is to reject our national policy.

We have all manner of ways to retaliate, but our ability to retaliate to some fanciful, "Strangelove-type" limited scenario is not the real question. The real question is how to keep it limited. If we cannot, then we come right back to the general exchange and we all know who the winners and losers are in such a fracas—no one. The bottom line is the same for all parties. Nuclear weapons are only weapons of deterrence. It is utter nonsense to talk about advantages of employment of nuclear weapons in an all-out war. The conclusion that MacArthur reached is the same that I have reached and that millions of our citizens are reaching all over this country: nuclear war has no meaning other than destruction and thus it is futile to pursue building up more of these weapons.

I will grant all of the opponents of this freeze that a technological breakthrough could change things. There is nothing in a nuclear freeze resolution that prohibits the Soviet Union or the United States from developing other weapons outside the nuclear sphere. We are not proposing a freeze on research and development of new weapons or new ideas which are nonnuclear. What we are proposing is to stop the development, testing and deployment of nuclear weapons in a verifiable and mutually agreed-upon mode. Believe me, I would like to ban all weapons of war, but that is naive. The pressing issue and the one we want to get at as soon as possible is the continuous buildup of nukes. Preceeding down the nuclear road any further has little prospect for either side. Once upon a time we had an advantage. We were the sole possessor of the bomb. It was a cheap way to go because we needed less men in uniform under the umbrella of the bomb. Now, there is no way we could have that kind of advantage again. We may pine for those good old days of the cold war, when we could literally "Bomb 'em back to the Stone Age," or we may postulate that we can cause the collapse of the Soviet economy with an all-out nuclear arms race. But even in times of great prosperity, that would be a foolish approach, not to mention attempting such an undertaking when there are difficult economic times. However, if we do not act now, we are certain, as Admiral Rickover predicted, to keep going down the path to oblivion. This is not a prediction based on cowardice nor is it throwing in the towel to communism. It is simply a fact of life—or death if you would so have it.

There is no question that we must be strong—very strong—in light of the way the Soviet Union conducts itself in the world. Our way, the free way, is the correct way—certainly not the suppressive, repressive totalitarianism which is the way of the Soviet Union. But there is no way for anyone to stand up to nukes, not for us, not for the Russians. The result of an accident or a miscalculation is megadeath and megadestruction, not to mention the effects on the total environment of our world. There will be no escape. Heroism and the will to stand and fight will be that of a mutual suicide.

Admiral Rickover said that after the great nuclear holocaust that is sure to come, there will probably be a new species to develop: one that would be smarter than we were. I am not enamored by the thought that my future world will be inhabited and governed by a bunch of intelligent cockroaches. If we are truly serious about stopping, reducing, and eliminating nuclear weapons, then we must take a serious look at the freeze proposal. The people want it, we want it, the Soviets say they want it. We may never know, if we do not make the offer. And, it just may be the best opportunity we will ever have.

Jonathan B. Bingham is a Congressman from the State of New York who is a principal sponsor of the nuclear freeze resolution in the House of Representatives.

There will be opponents of this resolution. They will say that it is not timely now. They will say we should wait. Wait until President Reagan has completed his arms buildup. Wait until the M-X, the B-1 bomber, and the Trident II submarine come on line. We may well ask, When will the time be more right than it is right now? Will the Russians stand still while we build the M-X, the B-1, and the Trident II? In fact, there is equality today. We are equally vulnerable, equally afraid, equally trapped. What we must work to avoid is the equality of extinction. The sense of fear and vulnerability is widespread. The people in Vermont and California feel it. The people in Germany, in Holland, and in Britain feel it. The people of the Soviet Union, I have no doubt, feel it. Only one group seems to be relatively untouched. It is that small group of world leaders upon whom the fate of the world rests. In the United States, the people are far ahead of their elected leaders. For years we have heard that the American people are uninterested in the question of nuclear destruction, that their eyes glaze over at the mention of nuclear terror, that a form of mass hypnosis has deadened the sensitivities of the American people to this most important issue. Now we see that it is not the people who are unconcerned. This movement for a nuclear freeze originated not in Washington, but at the grassroots—in cities and small towns across America. At town meetings and church suppers this movement was born. Those of us who are elected officials are only carrying out the clear desire of the public. The arms race must end and it must end now. This resolution will be referred to the Foreign Affairs Committee in the House. As a member of that committee, I pledge my best efforts to see that it is promptly considered by that committee and by the House as a whole.

James Armstrong is the United Methodist Bishop of Indiana, and also President of the National Council of Churches.

One of the most lethal nuclear weapons under production,

a Trident submarine, is to be called *Corpus Christi*—the body of Christ. That is an obscene blasphemy. Jesus Christ stands in direct contradiction to everything the nuclear arms race represents. A nuclear holocaust would incinerate this globe. It would turn it into a realm of insects and grass. The nuclear freeze resolution does not call for unilateral disarmament. The 32 member communions of the National Council of Churches do not call for unilateral disarmament. But there is a desperate need in such a day for unilateral initiatives, like that of Anwar Sadat when he flew from Cairo to Jerusalem to offer an olive branch. The time has come for the President Brezhnevs and the President Reagans of this world to turn aside from their predictable, partisan posturing, their public egos, and respond to the desperate need of the human family, that we may in time redeem the future for the family of humankind.

Ten years after the atomic bomb was dropped on Hiroshima in 1945, the science editor of the *New York Times* said that we had progressed so far in our development of nuclear weaponry that we had weaponry that would make that first atomic bomb sound like the pop of a toy pistol. And that was a quarter of a century ago. Now, in 1982, we are joining hands and spirits with persons around the world, hoping that we can avoid a thousand million hells exactly like that one in August 1945.

The National Council of Churches is an ecumenical organization that brings together some 32 member communions. Those member denominations, which range from Episcopal on one side to Baptist on the other, have each in their own way spoken on this theme, calling the nation back from undue reliance upon military violence. In November 1979 the governing board of the National Council, adding statement upon statement across the years from 1968 on, said something that is encapsulated in the Kennedy-Hatfield resolution. But it is not just those 32 member communions, not just the National Council of Churches. There seems to be a quickening conscience, perhaps belated, across the religious and moral community of humankind, that is responding to the urgent challenge of this hour. Pope John Paul II has called the arms race madness. The U.S. Conference of Catholic Bishops has courageously spoken of the course on which we are embarked. Two weeks ago, I lunched with Father Theodore Hesburgh, one of the great citizens of this nation, president of Notre Dame, who last November determined he would channel his considerable resources, energies, and capacities to dealing with this issue and this issue alone, and is now shuttling back and forth between Vienna and the United States, attempting to bring a measure of sanity to the public debate. Billy Graham, who has endorsed this resolution, said in a CBS interview in 1979: "The people of Russia want peace, the people of China want peace, the people of the United States want peace." Then he went on to use these two words: madness, insanity. He said: "I am for disarmament." It was not an irresponsible statement. Interestingly enough, his radio broadcast is called the "Hour of Decision"; and that is precisely where we are, and what we face. For religionists, scientists, physicians, those representing the media, students, this is our Hour of Decision. What will we do? In the various branches of our government, it is an Hour of Decision. And it is a fateful hour. But it is not just the fundamental institutions that we speak of; there are voices being heard everywhere across this country, in town meetings and in local congregations. I was talking with a young minister who, here in this city yesterday after his service, had petitions signed by his congregation relating to the nuclear freeze. That is happening. To read the array of scientific facts and projections is almost overwhelming. They suggest that we are poised at this moment at the abyss of Apocalypse Now. At the conclusion of his book *The Fate of the Earth*, Jonathan Schell writes: "One day—and it is hard to believe that it will not be soon—we will make our choice. Either we will sink into the final coma and end it all, or, as I trust and believe, we will awaken to the truth of our peril, a truth as great as life itself, and, like a person who has swallowed a lethal poison but shakes off his stupor at the last moment and vomits the poison up, we will break through the layers of our denials, put aside our fainthearted excuses, and rise up to cleanse the earth of nuclear weapons." The religious community must stand as one in the presence of this choice, this Hour of Decision. It goes back to the prophet's vision that foresaw the day when swords would be beaten into plowshares. Our Lord was born in a crude place, as an angel chorus sang about Peace on Earth. He came to be known as the Prince of Peace, saying, "Blessed are the peacemakers." And in the final hours of His life, when one took up a sword to defend him, Jesus told him to put away the sword, for those who live by the sword will perish by the sword. One of the truly great saints of this century, Albert Schweitzer, in a famous broadcast from Oslo many years ago, paraphrased those words, saying those who live by the bomb will perish by the bomb.

Reverend Timothy S. Healy, of the Society of Jesus, is President of Georgetown University in Washington, D.C.

I am happy to speak for the growing consensus in the Roman Catholic community worldwide. The profound reservation expressed in the Second Vatican Council about the use of nuclear weapons, and the even more serious reservation spoken by Pope John Paul II about the threat to use nuclear weapons, are about to become major issues within America's Catholic community. The dynamics have not yet made themselves fully felt, despite all their power and enormous reach. I am happy to support the nuclear freeze resolution, because I think it moves in the right direction. It is time we faced up to the folly of saying that the dichotomy is either "Red or dead." We could, for instance, get smart. We face a problem, but I think it is within the wisdom and the strength and the understanding of this nation to solve it.

When John Carroll founded Georgetown University 193 years ago, he referred in his letter to "this blessed Republic." It does not seem to me that "this blessed Republic" ought to be in the business of exterminating Russians or Chinese or itself. And let me add a personal note. Through some 30 years of teaching, I have seen three generations of kids I taught drafted, and have seen many of them killed. Every night when I am home at Georgetown I say Mass in Dahlgren Chapel for a group of students. We repeat the lovely prayer which begins:

> My peace I give you,
> My peace I leave unto you,

and it is for them that I pray for "peace in our day." As long as Americans are willing to sit back and imagine peace as a mysterious gift of God and thus do nothing about it, all of us are headed for trouble. When we grasp the invitation of that prayer, when we admit that peace is of our own making, of our own wits, of our own intelligence, of our own courage, we will have taken an enormous step forward. This resolution is just such a step.

Roger Mahony is Roman Catholic Bishop of the Diocese of Stockton, California.

I am speaking as an individual Catholic Bishop vitally interested in the moral dimensions of the current nuclear arms race. I gladly add my voice to the growing chorus of protests against the nuclear arms race because I believe the current arms policy of our nation, as well as of the Soviet Union, has long since exceeded the bounds of justice and moral legitimacy. Moreover, the nuclear arms race makes it impossible effectively to end the urgent crisis of world hunger. It can no longer be tolerated. Each day we permit it to continue without protest, it perpetuates itself by becoming embedded in our everyday habits and attitudes. What is needed, instead, is a radical change of our hearts and our attitudes—a new awareness of our calling to be a people dedicated to peace. Today, some 32 years and 50,000 nuclear weapons after the start of the nuclear arms buildup, the question of whether the use of nuclear weapons can be justified on any ethical grounds is rarely heard in our national debates and almost never in formal arms negotiations. All attention is riveted on questions such as how to put a ceiling on the further growth of weapons; for example, by limiting the number of warheads to no more than 10 per ICBM or 14 per sea-launched ballistic missile. It is the absence of this moral dimension in our public policy discussion and a growing moral callousness which permits some government officials to speak publicly and rashly of "limited" and "winnable" nuclear wars. This has impelled me to add my voice to the growing number of American Bishops who are calling for a fundamental about-face in the arms race. Recently we have heard public officials speak foolishly and imprudently of such "limited" and "winnable" nuclear wars, as if to prepare us to accept and accustom ourselves to such moral monstrosity. We have all become so numbed, so used to the nuclear umbrella, that we forget that less than a decade ago no responsible statesman, on either side, ever spoke of actually using nuclear weapons. With the present escalation in the nuclear arms race, there has also been an escalation in the rhetoric of threats and expectations and conceivable risks. The attitude that it is possible to "win" a nuclear war assumes that there is no longer any such thing as an unacceptable level of population loss. Any level of loss is apparently acceptable as long as our side "wins." In the face of such arrogance, such aridity of feeling and moral bankruptcy, we must not and cannot remain silent.

Just as the right to legitimate defense is not a justification for unleashing any and every form of destruction, so moral arguments for the possession of nuclear weapons for deterrence do not constitute support for every national arms policy that is advanced in the name of deterrence. The only possible Catholic support for a national nuclear deterrence policy depends on three related moral judgments: first, that the primary moral imperative is to prevent any use of nuclear weapons under any circumstances; secondly, that the possession of nuclear weapons is always an evil which could, at best, be tolerated, but only if the deterrence strategy is used in order to make progress on arms limitation and reductions; and thirdly, that the ultimate goal of what remains, at best, an interim deterrence policy is the eventual elimination of nuclear arms and of the threat of mutual assured destruction.

It is my judgment that the present United States and Soviet arms policy does not meet the demands of any of these three premises. Since I believe the American arms policy has exceeded the moral limits of deterrence and has eroded our real security, and since there has been up until now no serious connection between American arms policy and a serious attempt to reduce arms worldwide, it is my conviction that Catholics—and implicitly, all Americans—no longer have a secure moral basis to support actively or cooperate passively in the current U.S. arms policy and escalating arms race.

I am not advocating unilateral disarmament or an unqualified pacifism. But unilateral disarmament is something quite different from serious, persistent, even unilateral, initiatives toward bilateral disarmament. The goal must be disarmament, arms reduction, not merely a ceiling on new, even more monstrous weapons. I support a bilateral freeze by the U.S.A. and the USSR on all research, construction, or testing of new nuclear weapons systems. In addition, we must seriously consider a reduction of current nuclear armaments by one-half on both sides. I believe that this goal is both achievable and verifiable. In my judgment, nothing short of these two proposals will be adequate strategies for the present situation. We simply cannot continue on the course we are taking as a nation and as a people. Our future as American peoples, as Soviet peoples, as the human race on this planet, demands that we make a moral "about-face" on the nuclear arms race.

Rabbi Alexander M. Schindler is President of the Union of American Hebrew Congregations.

It is a privilege which I greatly appreciate to add my voice and to lend my strength to the effort which summons us. I speak not only for myself personally, but for the Union of American Hebrew Congregations, the national body of reformed Judaism in North America which I am privileged to lead. Last fall this congregational body, in convention assembled, adopted a resolution on the nuclear arms freeze and did so by an overwhelming majority—near unanimity, in fact. We are seized by the dread of a nuclear holocaust, and we find the proliferation of such weapons morally abhorrent. What kind of a ghoulish imagination is it which can project the possibility of a limited nuclear war, which can countenance the tactical use of such weapons, and even designate some of them as "clean"? There is nothing clean about a device which can put a torch to civilization; there are no possible limits to a nuclear conflict; there is no acceptable level of radioactive poisoning; there is nothing clean whatsoever about maimed limbs and burned flesh and broken spirits and widows' tears and a whole dark butchery without a soul. Let there be no doubt about it. The nuclear arms race is emerging as the central moral issue of our day. What Vietnam represented to the public conscience in the 1960s, the nuclear arms race will represent in the 1980s and in the 1990s. As religious leaders, we are resolved to lead this moral enterprise now as we led it successfully then. We are not the practioners of a "real-politik" or the pitchmen for the Pentagon; we are the spiritual descendants, the sons and the daughters, of the prophets. We serve the cause of life. We will continue to stand for sanity and reason, for compassion, and for peace.

Walter S. Wurzburger is Rabbi of Congregation Shaaray Tefila in Lawrence, New York, and President of the Synagogue Council of America.

Business cannot go on as usual in the face of the ominous threat to the very survival of mankind which is posed by the nuclear arms race. At a time when the superpowers possess nuclear arsenals sufficient not only to wipe out all civilization but to render the globe totally uninhabitable by human beings, it is the height of folly to develop ever deadlier weapons of destruction in a futile search for spurious security. Instead of increasing our margin of safety, they merely contribute to an ever more frightening balance of terror. Familiarity with the perils of nuclear proliferation must not breed indifference to the ever increasing threats to the very survival of mankind. It is our religious duty to appeal to all governments to embark on all-out efforts to halt the arms race and to bring about a mutual reduction of nuclear stockpiles. While unilateral disarmament would only invite aggression, bilateral progress in this direction would represent a giant step forward toward alleviation of hostility and tension. The nuclear arms race has drained enormous resources from the all-important task to battle against hunger, disease, and suffering. It is high time that we stop squandering energies on misguided efforts which, far from enhancing our security, only lead to the brink of unspeakable disaster. The religious community must muster the courage to fearlessly proclaim the message of the prophet Isaiah that "The earth was created to be settled"—not to witness the mass extinction of creatures bearing the image of God.

Richard Berendzen is President of American University in Washington, D.C., where President John F. Kennedy delivered a commencement address in 1963 announcing his dramatic proposal to ban the further testing of nuclear weapons. Nineteen years later, we traveled to American University to announce the Kennedy-Hatfield resolution for a nuclear weapons freeze. Dr. Berendzen recalled that moment of history in the following words.

According to widely heralded press accounts a few years ago, March 10, 1982, was allegedly to be the day of doom, the last day of earth. The thesis, basically, was that due to a chance alignment of planets, the sun would be disturbed, thereby triggering earthquakes on earth. Astronomers assured the public in the mid 1970's that those doomsday predictions were scientifically invalid. Yet other such predictions reasonably can be held by reasonable people. And ironically, their scientific explanation, too, comes from astrophysics—namely, from nuclear fusion. But their concerns are caused not by nature, but by humankind itself. And so it was on a sultry day nearly two decades ago, June 10, 1963, a young President of the United States, who had come to the American University to deliver the commencement speech, gave his historic address on nuclear weapons. At the outset of his speech, President Kennedy quoted John Masefield in his tribute to English universities: "There are few earthly things more beautiful than a university," and President Kennedy added, "His words are equally true here." He did not refer to spires and towers, to campus greens and ivy walls. He admired the splendid beauty of the university because it was a place where those who hate ignorance may strive to know, where those who perceive truth may strive to make others see. And then President Kennedy eloquently began the heart of his address: "I have therefore chosen this time and this place to discuss a topic on which ignorance too often abounds and the truth is too rarely perceived. Yet, it is the most important topic on earth—world peace. I am talking about genuine peace, not merely peace in our time. But peace for all time." Today, at a different time, but at the same place, a bipartisan group of Senators and Congressmen come to announce their proposals on this cardinal issue.

Randall Forsberg is the Director of the Institute for Defense and Disarmament Studies in Brookline, Massachusetts, and one of the founders of the nuclear freeze movement.

The National Committee of the Freeze Campaign, which represents participating groups and individuals around the country, has voted to endorse the Kennedy-Hatfield congressional resolution for a freeze and reductions of nuclear weapons. The campaign coordinators are delighted that mem-

bers of Congress have responded to growing popular concern
about the danger of nuclear war with a bipartisan proposal to
halt the arms race and reduce nuclear weapons. This congressional resolution follows a year of intense educational activity by freeze supporters around the nation. The freeze
campaign has focused popular anxiety about nuclear war on
the demand for an effective alternative to the arms race. The
campaign seeks a complete halt in the production of U.S. and
Soviet nuclear weapon systems as a minimal, first step toward
a global half in nuclear weapon production and the eventual
elimination of nuclear weapons. This nonpartisan demand
reaches across party lines and beyond politics as usual.
People feel deeply that whether we stop or continue the nuclear arms race is an issue of survival. As a result, thousands
of individuals not previously active in political movements
have volunteered to work for a nuclear weapon freeze. The
freeze proposal has been endorsed by more than 60 national
organizations and scores of prominent citizens from every
walk of life. Freeze resolutions have passed overwhelmingly
in the state legislatures of Connecticut, Massachusetts, and
Oregon and in the Houses of Wisconsin, Kansas, and New
York. In Vermont, 159 of 180 town meetings recently voted
for a freeze, as have town meetings and city and county
councils in South Dakota, Illinois, Indiana, Ohio, New
Hampshire, Maine, and Missouri. More than a million people
have signed freeze-related petitions. Popular referenda have
passed in parts of Massachusetts and Colorado; and initiatives
for statewide referenda have been launched in California,
Michigan, New Jersey, and Delaware. In all, freeze activities
are now underway in 43 states, with local groups organized
in two-thirds of the congressional districts.

The reason for this tremendous outpouring of support for a
nuclear weapons freeze is twofold. First, people have decided
that enough is enough. We have such enormous amounts of
nuclear overkill that the issue of who is "ahead" or "behind"
in the arms race has become meaningless. What is paramount
is to stop further developments on both sides. The United
States and the Soviet Union already have, between them,
about 50,000 nuclear weapons, while there are only 800 large
cities and towns in each country. The plans for this country
to produce 20,000 more nuclear warheads over the next decade (and the Soviet Union perhaps a like number) represent
an absurd waste of tax money sorely needed for national

economic recovery. Second, the next generation of nuclear weapons will dangerously increase the risk of nuclear war. Most of the new weapons are designed to attack nuclear forces and other military targets. In a crisis, the existence of such "counterforce" weapons will put pressure on the military on both sides to use their nuclear weapons before they are destroyed. To stop the race to oblivion before it becomes a reality is sensible and rational, but it will not be easy. It will take vision, courage, and hard work on the part of our national leaders.

Randall Kehler is National Coordinator of the Nuclear Weapons Freeze Campaign, headquartered in St. Louis; he is also one of the founders of the nuclear freeze movement.

In America today a rapidly growing number of people, from all walks of life, are educating themselves about the costs and dangers of the nuclear arms race. Seeking a way to move from education to action, thousands of people have joined together in a campaign to bring about a mutual U.S.-Soviet freeze on all nuclear weapons. We understand such a freeze to be an essential and veriable first step toward the reduction of nuclear weapons on both sides and, ultimately, the complete elimination of the threat of nuclear war. The Nuclear Weapons Freeze Campaign is broad-based and it is nonpartisan. It includes both conservatives and liberals, young and old, whites and nonwhites. While it has recently found an enthusiastic response in the halls of Congress, the campaign is rooted in town halls, union halls, and parish halls in hundreds of communities all across America.

The freeze proposal calls for a bilateral halt to the testing, production, and deployment of nuclear warheads, missiles, and other delivery systems. This is not simply an expression of general concern. It is a specific, concrete, and practical proposal. While there is no guarantee that the Soviets would automatically agree to a comprehensive freeze, our first objective, as American citizens, must be to persuade our own government to initiate such a proposal, taking full advantage of the democratic processes which we in this country are fortunate to have.

The freeze proposal rests on a number of basic premises. First, we are convinced that nuclear war, even a so-called "limited" or "theater" nuclear war, whether caused by accident or design, would cause a level of death and destruction unprecedented in human history and, possibly, the termination of all life on this planet. Second, we are also convinced that the real reductions in nuclear weapons which we all seek—reductions not just in one category of weapons but in the overall nuclear arsenals of both sides—will not come about unless preceded by a comprehensive, bilateral freeze as a minimal first step. Third, we see the overall nuclear arsenals of the U.S. and the Soviet Union as roughly equal, with obvious and inevitable advantages and disadvantages on both sides with regard to particular weapons systems. This rough equality offers an historic and unprecedented opportunity for freezing the nuclear arms race where it is, without either side thereby gaining a significant advantage. Fourth, we believe that it would be a grave mistake for the U.S. to proceed with its planned new generation of nuclear weapons systems. If these new systems are produced and deployed, they will upset the overall balance of nuclear forces which now exists. They will greatly destabilize the already precarious restraints on both sides. They will significantly increase the problems of detection and verification, making future arms control agreements far more difficult. And, instead of providing the Soviets an incentive to halt the nuclear arms race, these new U.S. weapons systems will most assuredly give the Soviets an incentive to go forward with their own generation of new weapons systems. Fifth, the bilateral freeze we are proposing, because it is so comprehensive—covering the testing and production as well as the deployment of both countries' nuclear weapons—would be highly verifiable. Indeed, it would be more verifiable than most previous arms control agreements between the U.S. and the Soviet Union. Sixth, and lastly, we regard the world's preparations for nuclear war as a tragic waste of human and natural resources desperately needed for life-affirming rather than life-destroying purposes.

Because the bilateral freeze proposal is so inherently clear and comprehensible, because it makes so much common sense, it is winning the support of a wide spectrum of the American people. Though the campaign is scarcely one year old, already more than a million Americans have signed freeze-related petitions. Twenty-three city councils, including those in Fort Wayne, Indiana; Youngstown, Ohio; Cleveland; Baltimore; and St. Louis, have endorsed the freeze. County boards of supervisors in Pitkin County, Colorado; Alameda County, California; Franklin County, Massachusetts; Montgomery County, Maryland; and Loudon County, Virginia have also endorsed the freeze. More than 250 town meetings in Vermont, New Hampshire, and Maine have voted—in most cases overwhelmingly—to support the freeze. Freeze resolutions have been adopted by the New York State Assembly, the House of Representatives in Kansas and in Wisconsin, and by both houses of the state legislature in Connecticut, Oregon, Massachusetts, Vermont, Maine, and Minnesota. The freeze has already won decisive referendum victories in western Massachusetts and Boulder, Colorado, and there are efforts underway to put the freeze on the ballot statewide in New Jersey, Delaware, and Michigan, and in California, a state which comprises 10 percent of the U.S. population. In addition, the freeze has been publicly endorsed by more than 60 national and international organizations, and by hundreds of nationally prominent individuals from every sector of our society, including every major religious denomination in America. The campaign is now active in 43 states and 279 congressional districts. And it is only just beginning.

There can be no doubt that a comprehensive, bilateral freeze on the nuclear arms race is an idea whose time has come. For too long the American people have been silent on this issue, while government leaders and military experts, in the name of national security, have brought us ever closer to the edge of nuclear annihilation. Now, finally, the American people are saying, in ever-increasing numbers and with ever-increasing impatience, "This madness must cease! In the name of our common humanity, the nuclear arms race must be stopped, and then reversed!"

John Smith is Mayor of Prichard, Alabama; he is also a member of the Alabama Conference of Black Mayors.

The Alabama Conference of Black Mayors endorses the resolution on the nuclear arms freeze, based on, first, the senseless stalemate position which we have come to with respect to the use of such weapons by the Soviet Union and the United States against each other; second, the moral and verified reality that a nation which prides itself on the wealth of knowledge and high technology should not continue to utilize its wisdom and the great energy of the federal government, terrorized by Soviet threats, to plan for nuclear war. We have come to a civilized position as a nation, and to continue on this course of nuclear buildup is senseless. Third, we endorse the idea that the related defense operations in our state and their possibility of being target areas is an issue of concern to us. Fourth, we believe that during this period of international economic crisis, we should begin to establish an expanded basis for economic cooperation, and cultural understanding and cultural appreciation of each other. Neither the Soviet Union nor the United States can afford to neglect its economy and resource needs of its citizens and to continue the traditional military defense and foreign policy positions against each other.

While reading the position statements released by many of our leaders throughout the years on this subject, it is as though we have built up a tremendous literature of propaganda, until now its feedback has started to impact on us. To continue in this course simply means that cities such as ours will be hurt. The Alabama Conference of Black Mayors, which is the largest membership conference of black mayors in the United States, has 23 members who believe this course will only have a negative impact on trying to build a viable economy for our cities. We have organized, it seems, a reactionary negative foreign policy and defense strategy, rather than a forward, positive purpose to achieve good works throughout our world environment. The Alabama Conference of Black Mayors endorses the idea of a nuclear freeze because of the emphasis on prevention, and supports an emphasis on a purposeful foreign policy and defense strategy, based on economic stability and development opportunities. This will result, we believe, in greater opportunity for the 23 cities represented by our organization.

As Mayor of the City of Prichard, my concerns are for the enormous number of people left in the dark on this issue. We have largely limited debate and discussion on this subject to the intelligent, the educated, and the well-off. Those large segments of the poor, such as the city of Prichard, are not involved. We are a coastal zone city; we are situated near a major port; we are situated near a defense-related industry; we are situated near the planned Tombigbee Waterway and a major university center. I am told that these are prime nuclear attack areas. If we are part of a region that may be a

target, we should be more intricately and continuously involved in these discussions. I am concerned for the young
people in our community who are not exposed to this issue,
but will be expected to live with it and, more importantly,
lack the overall public education and knowledge of the realities of a nuclear war. I strongly recommend that you consider
providing for public education and public awareness forums,
so that more people at the grass-roots level can support and
become actively involved in this movement. I believe that this
will result in the necessary knowledge and competence on the
part of our people to understand this vital issue, the ethics
involved in it, the technology involved in it, and to speak out
very forcefully and directly on this issue and support it.

I would like to invite you to hold meetings in the community. It would serve a great good if you can channel these
types of energies in cities such as Prichard, and involve public officials, business leaders, citizens, the medical profession,
and our cable television system. Federal government officials,
our congressional liaison officers, could play a vital role in
educating our population and utilizing our resources at the
local level to help elevate this cause. We must continue this
great effort, for it will define the ethical, economic, and technological future of the United States.

H. Jack Geiger is professor of community medicine at City
College of New York and a member of Physicians for Social
Responsibility.

For more than three decades scientific and medical groups
have been warning of the danger of nuclear weapons. It is
more than 20 years since physicians first studied the effects of
a single modern nuclear weapon on a modern city and
showed that it would be an event with millions of deaths and
millions of injuries, almost beyond comprehension, and certainly without parallel in the past history of the species. It is
more than 30 years since Albert Einstein, at the dawn of the
age of nuclear weaponry, said that everything has changed
except the way we think. As scientists we know the almost in-
comprehensible power of these weapons—their power to
crush, burn, poison, and destroy the environment. As physicians, we know that we face the final epidemic, that even a
so-called limited nuclear confrontation would involve death,

devastation, disease, and disaster, the return of plague, of epidemic, tuberculosis, of malnutrition, and genetic malformation. Yet during these decades the hands on the atomic clock, if anything, have moved steadily closer to the apocalypse. A single M-X missile carries the death and destructive capacity of 1600 Hiroshima weapons. And the M-X missile and its Soviet counterparts are good symbols, because they force on both of us the requirement for billions of dollars of expenditure on them, while we cut school lunches and turn our backs on the health of our children and our elderly. We become societies that shelter our weapons like treasures and expose our children to hunger and neglect. I see the nuclear freeze resolution as a critical first step in scientific terms, in medical terms, above all in human terms as a way of turning away from the apocalypse instead of rushing toward it. I support the Kennedy-Hatfield resolution as consistent with an earlier piece of important legislation. It is a kind of New Endangered Species Act. Only this time the endangered species is all mankind.

Vera Morkovin is a surgeon and is associate professor and chief of the division of emergency medicine at the University of Illinois; she is also a member of Physicians for Social Responsibility.

The most personal reaction I have of what I have learned about the possibilities of nuclear war is the fear of trying to consider myself as a physician trying to treat the patients who would be victims of such a conflagration. In Hiroshima, we saw not only the total destruction in areas where people died instantly, but the feeble attempts of the surviving medical personnel to treat the horrible injuries that resulted from firestorms, the thermal effect of nuclear weapons, the blast effect, and the radiation effect. The three means by which nuclear weapons cause the greatest damage are the blast, thermal, and radiation effects. The organization which I represent, Physicians for Social Responsibility, started out by trying to study and inform ourselves about the actual medical effects of nuclear war; we finally reached the conclusion that these medical effects are so great it is impossible for the medical profession to respond in any adequate way; we have characterized this concept as the final epidemic. A few examples: 11 miles away from the center of a one-megaton blast, all glass would break; the fragments would be flying at 100 miles an hour, as missiles aimed at all vulnerable human bodies in their path. I think of the blast injuries resulting from the explosion, and I think of the fractures and the ruptured spleens and the crushed brains, and it is not a pretty thought. I am particularly concerned about the thermal effects. In this country today, we have only about 2000 burn units in hospitals, because burns require very special treatment nurses around the clock, and sophisticated medical facilities. Obviously, in the survival areas surrounding a nuclear blast, medical facilities will be totally unavailable. The number of burn victims predicted from a one-megaton explosion would fill all the burn units in this country many times over. The idea of shelters is propounded by some government officials; in the past, even in conventional war in Europe, some shelters proved to be crematoria rather than safe places; in a nuclear war, even deep underground shelters could immediately burn up all the people in those shelters. Radiation injuries can kill many, many people very rapidly. The people in Hiroshima who died between two and four weeks after the bomb were those who had received fatal doses of radiation. The radiation would be carried 20 miles downwind by a single megaton bomb; it has been estimated that the people who were exposed to that radiation over a period of 12 to 24 hours would be receiving something like 3500 rems; a rem is a unit of radiation, and 300 to 400 are considered fatal in most cases. They would receive nine to ten times the fatal dose. The island of Bikini, which was 18 miles from the nuclear test in 1954, is still considered uninhabitable and will be so for 30 to 40 years because of the amount of radiation. I cannot believe that there is any such thing as a limited nuclear war. To me that is as inconceivable as being "a little bit pregnant." The lack of hospitals and doctors and medical facilities will be totally and completely crippled and will be made even worse by the electromagnetic pulse effect, which will knock out all of the electronic equipment upon which we depend so much in modern medicine. If it were possible that only one area of the world would be totally destroyed and that fairly large areas would manage to survive, then the later effects have to be considered, such as the nitrogen and oxygen combinations caused by thermonuclear explosions; these compounds would rise and destroy a large percentage of the ozone layer. Realistically, what does this mean from a medical standpoint? The ozone layer protects us from ultraviolet radiation from the sun. With only half of the ozone layer destroyed, people going out in the sunlight would receive blistering sunburns immediately, and the possibility of plant growth and animal life would be greatly limited. Thirty-five miles from a one-megaton explosion, everyone with their eyes open would be blinded. Animal life as well as human life would be blinded. Our public health system, as we know it now, would be gone; we take for granted the fact that we are protected by our advanced technology from epidemics. With that system gone, with widespread insect vectors which can survive radiation much better than mammals, with the uncontrolled growth of animal life, we would be swamped with epidemics such as typhus, cholera, plague, and so on. We cannot even conceive of the health hazard to hundreds of thousands of workers. The psychological consequences, which are also medical effects, are serious ones we cannot predict. A close friend of mine, who was present at the Hyatt Hotel when the balcony fell, was wading ankle-deep in blood trying to rescue some of the people in that catastrophe; he almost suffered a temporary mental breakdown. The effect on the rescue workers was so great that they all needed psychiatric care. We do not know whether the rescue personnel would be doctors or would be able to function at anything like the greatest efficiency in the face of the awful destruction of a nuclear war. Finally, I am concerned about the psychological effects now, before the possibility of such a conflagration, on our people. We have all alluded to the fact that there seems to have been apathy about this issue until very recently. One of our psychiatrists coined the phrase "psychic numbing." I know that I personally, and most of my friends and colleagues and family, were victims of psychic numbing up until recently. We couldn't bring ourselves to talk about this horror. Now that we have started to talk about it, I must say that many physicians involved in the group that I am working with are beginning to feel differently. Physicians for Social Responsibility is one of the most rapidly growing medical organizations in the country today. It has doubled its membership to about 10,000 members within one year. Physicians are not notably concerned about progressive or liberal political causes. In fact, most of my colleagues have been traditionally conservative medical practitioners. The community I live in is that type of community, and yet we have been asked to present a grand round on nuclear war at one of our local hospitals. We need more medical education. Physicians for Social Responsibility, in collaboration with the Council for a Livable World, has sponsored 17 symposia in the past year and a half in major cities throughout the country. These symposia are drawing medical personnel; they are accredited for continuing medical education, which all physicians are required to take. In other words, we are learning about the great dangers of a nuclear epidemic. It is medical policy, when we are confronted with an incurable disease or one which we cannot hope to do anything about after it occurs, to turn to the area of preventive medicine. I think physicians are beginning to see this. Physicians for Social Responsibility is affiliated with a worldwide organization, International Physicians for the Prevention of Nuclear War, which involves many countries. The American Medical Association recently passed a resolution to inform the President and Congress of the medical consequences of nuclear war, to educate physicians and the public, because the available data revealed there is no adequate medical response to a nuclear holocaust. I would like to read you one short quotation from one of the physicians who attended the international conference of Physicians for the Prevention of Nuclear War in April 1981: "We physicians, as the professional group that is the most influential in the struggle for the life and health of all the people in the world and the most knowledgeable about the tragic consequences of nuclear war, can make a bigger contribution to the cause to prevent it. Our patients trust us; they entrust their health and their lives to us. And in keeping with our professional honor, in keeping with the Oath of Hippocrates, we have no right to hide from them the danger to their lives that now threatens us all. Today, physicians working all over the world must regard the struggle against the danger of nuclear war to be not only the duty of an honest humanitarian person, but also a professional duty. This must be understood by the World Health Organization. We are dealing not with political problems but with the preservation of the health and lives of all people."

That statement, to which almost every physician whom I know would subscribe, was made by the Soviet cardiologist who is Brezhnev's personal physician. Shortly after that meeting, when he went back to the Soviet Union, a nationwide television program on the dangers of nuclear war from the medical point of view was broadcast to 150 million Soviet citizens. There is danger for both sides, but I think that physicians, medical people, and scientists can unite, so that this worldwide move toward a freeze has some possibility of being realized.

Jerome Grossman is President of the Council for a Livable World; he is also President of the Committee for a Nuclear Weapons Freeze, organized in Wellesley, Massachusetts.

If you visit the John F. Kennedy Memorial Library at Columbia Point in south Boston, Massachusetts, you will see a film about the Partial Nuclear Test Ban, the most successful treaty ever negotiated between the U.S. and the Soviet Union. This treaty, signed and ratified in 1963, banned nuclear weapons tests in the atmosphere, in outer space, and under water. Kennedy was President at the time. Remarkably, this agreement came into force less than one year after the superpowers confronted each other in the Cuban missle crisis, which almost ended in nuclear war. The treaty is still in full force. The film shows a scene in early 1963. John Kennedy looks silently out of the window of the Oval Office. It is raining. A voice is heard, the voice of Jerome Wiesner recalling the event. Wiesner was Science Adviser to the President. He is now the retired president of M.I.T. Wiesner tells his story: "I remember one day when he asked me what happens to the radioactive fallout, and I told him it was washed out of the clouds by the rain. And he said, looking out of the window, 'You mean it's in the rain out there?' and I said, 'Yes.' He looked out the window, very sad, and didn't say a word for several minutes." What was John Kennedy thinking of? Of his children, Caroline and John? Of his own lost childhood? Of his mortality?

President Kennedy could have found experts on both sides of this question. The dangers to human health of fallout were minimized and even denied by many in those days. Were we fortunate that Wiesner was there? Or did the President make the decision out of his own visceral reaction? You don't have to be an expert to have your say on public policy. You go with whatever level of information you have. For too long, the American people, the Russian people, and indeed all the peoples of this earth have been intimidated by the military technocrats on nuclear weapons policies. These fateful questions have been monopolized by the strategists and designers of military hardware. They have created their own language and developed their lunatic scenarios of such complexity that the mere citizen feels excluded from the debate.

We cannot allow this situation to continue. The nature and effects of nuclear weapons are not beyond the grasp of most people. The basic issues of catastrophe and survival are well within the capacities of the average citizen. The technical details of the awful weapons are not the keys to basic policy. The problem is not the hardware. It is the doctrine and behavior surrounding nuclear weapons. Like President Kennedy, we must restore our gut reactions to a place of honor. We must not suppress our instinctive revulsion and moral outrage to these games of death. We must prevent the technocrats from playing with our survival. As a congenital optimist, I refuse to be swept by the tide of helplessness as we move from hard talk to hardware, from negotiations to confrontation. As an organizer of people, I know that change is driven by moral outrage; anger wedded to our sense of right and wrong. The late Justice William O. Douglas wrote in his autobiography that at the very start of his career on the Supreme Court, Charles Evans Hughes, then Chief Justice, told him, "You must remember one thing. At the constitutional level where we work, ninety percent of any decision is emotional. The rational part of us supplies the reasons for supporting our predilections."

I am morally outraged at any plans to drop nuclear bombs on people for any reason. I am morally outraged that the United States and the Soviet Union have continued to develop ever more horrible variations of nuclear weapons. I am morally outraged at the Soviet Union and the United States for joining in the insane arms race. In my hometown of Wellesley, Massachusetts, the members of the Nuclear Freeze Committee express their moral outrage. We think globally but act locally. We help people to move in steady progression from information to fear to outrage to hope to demands for action. And the greatest of these is hope. We believe in the power of public opinion, everywhere. In America it may be expressed within the traditions of western liberalism. In the Soviet Union it may require popular and working-class revolts, as in Poland and Hungary and the Ukraine. But in the long run public opinion will not be denied.

The knowledge about the dangers to civilization and even to survival is the most important message brought by the nuclear freeze movement. There is an important link between the education of the public to the awful truth about nuclear war and the setting of public policy. Any administration or any Congress which believes that it can continue to trust to luck, that it can continue to muddle through the precarious situation, especially that it can even play politics with human survival, is making an irresponsible and terrible mistake. The nuclear freeze movement is grateful to Senators Kennedy and Hatfield as well as their cosponsors for formally recognizing the crisis and responding to it with their congressional resolution. But this is only the beginning. The knowledge is out: not only the technology of how to make a nuclear bomb, but also the knowledge of its effects. The knowledge is combined with feeling; moral outrage wedded to an intense love of our planet and our species. From now on we will not be dissociated from the central fact of our time; we must rescue ourselves.

George W. Ball is Senior Managing Director of Lehman Brothers in New York City; he served as Under Secretary of State in the administrations of President Kennedy and President Johnson.

The Kennedy-Hatfield resolution is an effort to impress on Congress and the American people that unless we change our current nuclear policy we have little hope of avoiding a nuclear catastrophe beyond all human imaginings. Our government's approach to nuclear weapons has, for a long while, been unrealistic—reflecting the speculations of nuclear theoreticians whose logic chopping has been used to justify an accelerating nuclear arms race. Now we are approaching the point of no return.

In government circles, one hears increasing expressions of dangerous nonsense which thoughtful men and women had ruled out years ago—that we should regard nuclear bombs as potential weapons of war and not merely of deterrence, and prepare our tactics accordingly; that short- or medium-range missiles could be fired without necessarily triggering a full-scale nuclear exchange; that, if we were all to burrow like moles under the ground, many of us could still survive a nuclear way (though why anyone would want to is by no means clear); and finally, that, as the Vice-President himself has said, nuclear wars may be "winnable."

Meanwhile we pursue the false god of nuclear equality (which for all too many means nuclear superiority), demonstrating by dubious sleight-of-hand with numbers that we are dangerously far behind in nuclear arms. Some even look through a "window of vulnerability" as through a glass darkly. The scholastics have devised a vocabulary of their own which obscures thought more than expresses it; not only does that vocabulary need careful scrutiny, but we must challenge the intentions of the speakers. When administration officials proclaim that arms control negotiations should be postponed until we have achieved "a position of strength," they rule out all hope of controlling the arms race, for the Soviets will certainly keep pace with any nuclear breakthroughs—advancing the art and creating new systems to the point where all control becomes impossible.

Though the administration's statements and policies may not scare the Soviets, they certainly frighten our friends. Our European allies are more and more questioning the leadership of a nation whose government seems addicted to a rhetoric even more bellicose than the Soviets' and which seems hypnotized by an ellusive "equality." For better or worse, the sensitivity of Europe to the statements and actions of our government has always been a dominating fact of the Western alliance—a fact that we dare not ignore. Thus we cannot avoid considerable responsibility for the demonstrations in European streets against the implantation of Pershings and cruise missiles on European soil. These demonstrations were temporarily halted when the administration reluctantly began negotiations on this limited area of nuclear policy—but that is only the beginning of the story. As warm weather returns, so will the demonstrators and they will continue to gain in noise and number until we begin prompt and serious negotiations to turn back the nuclear arms race all across the board. Do not expect rational argument from the demonstrators.

Aware that Europe has little role in shaping nuclear policy and that their fate is in the hands of an American government that pursues a persistently confrontational course, many young Europeans are turning from logic to emotion, opting, in frustration, for the suicidal policy of unilateral disarmament.

Though European protests have served as forerunners of organized protests just getting under way in America, American expressions of concern have so far been remarkably responsible. Americans are becoming more and more concerned at the insensitivity our government has shown toward the nuclear issue. The people are waking up. Americans are famous for common sense and, though increasing numbers are becoming aware of the slippery slope down which we are sliding, they have avoided the irrational excesses manifested in Europe. I know no American who would save himself or herself at the cost of freedom. Yet let us not be too complacent; if America does not soon embark on a serious and realistic arms reduction negotiation, and if our government officials continue to suggest, by word or action, that nuclear bombs are a potential weapon of war, the national outcry may ultimately take a more strident and less responsible form.

That is the significance of the Kennedy-Hatfield resolution. It gives responsible expression to our imperative need to clear the air of a deceptive dialectical fog. It rejects the contention that we dare negotiate only from what the nuclear pundits call "strength"—which serves as an excuse for not negotiating at all. It provides a sensible alternative to continuing the arms race to the point where the advent of increasingly complex and elaborate new weapons systems will destroy the possibility of verification and thus close off our last clear chance for effective negotiation. It expresses also our need to break free from the deceptive tyranny of numbers and from the metaphysicians who manipulate those numbers, and to find a new form of negotiation through which serious progress toward arms reduction can be achieved.

By seeking an agreement with the Soviet Union to "achieve a mutual and verifiable freeze on the testing, production, and further deployment of nuclear warheads, missiles, and other delivery systems," the United States would quickly reestablish the confidence of its allies now so tragically waning. Even more important, it would restore the faith of rational men and women that our government is earnestly striving to save mankind from its own self-destruction. But though a freeze is an essential first step, its major value lies in providing a starting point for the more fundamental process of phased nuclear arms reduction.

Our disappointing experience has clearly demonstrated that reductions of any significance or magnitude cannot be achieved under a system such as has been used in the SALT negotiations. Under that system the negotiators seek vainly to establish equivalencies of weapons systems—of their warheads, throw-weights, and other recondite attributes—that in the nature of things cannot be equated. In such an effort, each side is the victim of its own competing vested interests. Each of the American services—the Army, the Navy, the Air Force—fights for a larger part of the turf, a greater share in the design and management of nuclear weapons. Each pushes hard for its own weapons system with the support of its own nuclear metaphysicians and engages in reciprocal back-scratching to achieve that end. If SALT II proved anything, it was that a negotiation seeking to satisfy all competitive interests is totally unsuited to achieving effective reductions. After American negotiators have accommodated all these competing baronies and developed a negotiating position complete with fallbacks, they will have jettisoned all possibility of serious progress toward arms reduction.

But how can we avoid negotiating from a base that reflects the collective demands of all the parties involved? America has already developed and successfully demonstrated the answer in our trade negotiations. We must stop trying to measure system against system, throw-weight against throw-weight, and embark on a series of phased, across-the-board percentage reductions. Of course, that will upset the theoreticians; such a procedure, they will say, would produce serious distortions and inequalities. One country might end up with more weapons than another in one or more weapons systems. But even in a negotiation based on across-the-board percentage reductions, there could be some room for adjusting the most outrageous disequilibria. In any event, that should not prove crucial. Each side already possesses such a massive amount of overkill that a numerical parity in warheads or throw-weight or even qualitative advantage loses most of its relevance. As one wise man recently observed, numbers of nuclear weapons would be important were we dealing in tens but they have little relevance when dealing in thousands.

Today the nuclear arms race is not only speeding out of

control but out of all possibility of control. One hears talk in Washington circles of casting overboard the few notable achievements of past negotiations: for example, not renewing the ABM Treaty barring antiballistic missiles. Given the momentum of technological development, sooner or later there will be pressure to abolish the agreement barring weapons from outer space.

It is already late in the day, but we can still interrupt and reverse the nuclear weapons process. Our generation may be the last one offered the chance to shackle the monster that could destroy us all. It is not a chance responsible men and women can neglect.

Paul Warnke served as Director of the U.S. Arms Control and Disarmament Agency in the Carter administration; he was the chief negotiator of the United States on the SALT II Treaty with the Soviet Union, and he is also a member of the Committee for National Security.

The Committee for National Security is a citizens group dedicated to the genuine security of the United States. We want to voice our support for the call for a United States-Soviet Union nuclear weapons freeze. It is one of the most meaningful steps that could be taken to revitalize the nuclear arms control process, to halt the nuclear arms race, and to put us in a position to negotiate substantial and continuing mutual reductions. Together with the other members of the committee, I urge the Congress to support the nuclear freeze resolution and to call upon the President to carry it out, both in letter and in spirit. Now, we will be told that this sort of move sends the wrong signal to the Soviets. But I submit there are better ways to communicate with the Soviet Union than by building up more and more and more and more dangerous weapons. There is, for example, the bargaining table. There we can communicate in a fashion that will lead to greater security. We are now living on borrowed time, all of us. I recognize that there are international problems of great importance. But they must not be allowed to obscure the urgency of this issue, or the gravity of the danger to our survival. I would like to quote from Andrei Sakharov, whose own personal sacrifice, whose own dissent against Soviet internal repression, gives him special credentials. He wrote the following back in 1975: "The unchecked growth of thermonuclear arsenals and the buildup toward confrontation threaten mankind with the death of civilization and physical annihilation. The elimination of that threat takes unquestionable priority over all other problems in international relations." I think that Andrei Sakharov would join us in supporting the nuclear freeze.

Thomas D. Davies is a Rear Admiral, now retired, in the United States Navy; he is a former Commander of U.S. Carrier Divisions of the Atlantic Fleet and the Mediterranean Fleet. He is also a former Chief of Naval Development in the Department of Defense and a former Assistant Director of the U.S. Arms Control and Disarmament Agency.

I speak of course as a private citizen. I will try to express my views on nuclear weapons as they relate to national defense. These views are based upon almost 30 years of active service in the Navy, at sea and ashore and in both operational and technical fields. My experience also covers 7 years in the arms control area, including chairing two negotiating delegations and several National Security Council committees supporting and coordinating negotiations.

The unfolding events since the advent of the nuclear bomb has made it clear that these devices cannot be dealt with as ordinary weapons. The self-penalties for their use are such as to make clear to everyone that use of these devices can only be contemplated in retaliation for such use against us. In other words their utility is as a deterrent to our adversary using them against us. The circular argument that results from this is that the Soviets are deterring us and we are deterring them—a situation that benefits no one but the people who participate in or write about this standoff.

In spite of the astronomical numbers used to express their energy release—and their cost—it is clear to me that any way to exploit these devices to gain advantage for the United States evaporated long ago—with the advent of the Soviet bomb, to be specific. Thus their existence and continued development gains us nothing, and the risks of their inadvertent use and their cost in dollars, manpower, and talents are of sizable proportions.

Under these circumstances it seems clear that the only rational approach is arms control—that is by the negotiation of verifiable agreements for a mutual freeze and major reductions, to eliminate the endless increases in the numbers of warheads in the U.S. and Soviet inventories. Thirty-odd years ago, inventories were measured in tens; today they are measured in tens of thousands, and our national security and our ability to influence world events in our interest have not been enhanced.

The Kennedy-Hatfield resolution seems to me to call for the only rational approach to nuclear weapons. I believe it to be in the national security interest of the United States. Certainly the objective of the U.S. should be to attempt to stop the open-ended increases of these dangerous weapons, on a mutual basis with the USSR.

Herbert Scoville, Jr., is a former Deputy Director of the Central Intelligence Agency for Research (Science and Technology); he is also a former Assistant Director of the U.S. Arms Control and Disarmament Agency.

A freeze on the testing, production, and deployment of strategic weapons systems can be verified, so that we can be confident that any violation that would significantly affect our security would have a high probability of being detected. Satisfactory verification does not require that any violation, no matter how insignificant, has to be detected, as some who wish to foreclose any arms control agreement would like the public to believe. As Paul Nitze has testified, verification capabilities should be tailored to the security significance of any violation.

In a freeze, certain elements would have a better probability of detection than others. For example, the production of new missiles is harder to monitor with high confidence than their testing and deployment, which can be verified relatively easily by national technical means, which is another word for technical intelligence. Thus, some uncertainty in production can be corrected by information on the other two phases of the weapons cycle.

Furthermore, a freeze would mean a stop to all activities in any weapons program, so that the detection of even one new missile or aircraft would be evidence of a violation. This simplifies the verification over that required for monitoring a ceiling. Thus, a ceiling on deployed cruise missiles might be very hard to monitor, but a total ban on their production and deployment could be verified with high confidence, because the detection of even one missile would be enough to prove a violation.

For both nuclear warhead testing and fissionable materials production, procedures for verification have been already worked out. The Comprehensive Test-Ban Treaty negotiators have agreed on verification arrangements, which include unmanned seismic stations and invitational on-site inspections. Since both the U.S. and USSR have hundreds of thousands of kilograms of weapons-grade fissionable material, it is hard to see how any clandestine production that could significantly add to these stockpiles could escape detection by our intelligence.

Big reductions of strategic arms can also be verified. The standing consultative commission after SALT I agreed on ways to monitor the destruction of existing strategic delivery vehicles. Procedures were also worked out and tested in the 1960s for withdrawing and transferring to peaceful programs fissionable material from existing warheads without compromising weapons design information. Of course, any agreement on deep reductions would, to be meaningful, have to include provisions to prevent replacement by new weapons, so the verification would have to include many of the arrangements for a freeze.

In sum, the key elements of any freeze or reduction agreement that might be negotiated can be adequately verified without a requirement for intrusive and unacceptable procedures. The SALT treaties have already set precedents for solving many of the detailed problems that might arise.

Verification can no longer be legitimately used as an excuse for not proceeding with a freeze and reductions agreement. I believe that a freeze on the testing, production, and deployment of nuclear weapons and delivery systems, leading to deep reductions, as expressed in the Kennedy-Hatfield resolution, is a sound arms control measure which can lead to a greater security for all peoples.

George F. Kennan is Professor Emeritus at the Institute for Advanced Study in Princeton, New Jersey, and a former U.S. Ambassador to the Soviet Union. He is also one of the

most respected experts of our time in foreign policy. Earlier
this year, he endorsed the nuclear freeze resolution in these
words: "Progress along the lines of the Kennedy-Hatfield
resolution is absolutely imperative and urgent. It can no longer be delayed and it should supersede all partisan and self-
serving considerations." On May 19, 1981, the Einstein
Foundation awarded the Albert Einstein Peace Prize to Ambassador Kennan for his noteworthy contributions over many
years to the prevention of nuclear war. In accepting the prize,
he delivered a brilliant essay on the human condition in the
nuclear age.

A person would have to be wholly insensitive, or perhaps
selfless to the point of saintliness, in order not to be moved
by such an honor as the Einstein Foundation is conferring on
me today. I am neither of those things; so I am naturally
deeply grateful and appreciative. On the other hand, I cannot
help but have my doubts as to whether I have fully deserved
it. And for that reason I can look on it only as a mark of
confidence and of encouragement—encouragement to myself
and to a great many other people—encouragement to continue to do what little may be in our power to assure that we
of this generation, here and elsewhere, do not, in deference to
our military fears, commit the supreme sacrilege of putting
an end to the civilization out of which we have grown, the
civilization which has made us what we are, the civilization
without which our children and grandchildren can have no
chance for self-realization, possibly no chance of life itself.

This, as I see it, is the task to which the Einstein Foundation has devoted itself. Beside it, all personal considerations
ought to fade into insignificance. I am grateful for the opportunity to associate myself publicly with this cause. And I am
grateful for the admonition which the award implies: the admonition to neglect nothing—no effort, no unpleasantness, no
controversy, no sacrifice—which could conceivably help to
preserve us from committing this fatal folly.

What can we do?

Adequate words are lacking to express the full seriousness
of our present situation. It is not just that we are for the moment on collision course politically with the Soviet Union,
and that the process of rational communications between the
two governments seems to have broken down completely; it is
also—and even more importantly—the fact that the ultimate

sanction behind the conflicting policies of these two governments is a type and volume of weaponry which could not possibly be used without utter disaster for us all.

For over 30 years, wise and far-seeing people have been warning us about the futility of any war fought with nuclear weapons and about the dangers involved in their cultivation. Some of the first of these voices to be raised were those of great scientists, including outstandingly that of Albert Einstein himself. But there has been no lack of others. Every President of this country, from Dwight Eisenhower to Jimmy Carter, has tried to remind us that there could be no such thing as victory in a war fought with such weapons. So have a great many other eminent persons.

When one looks back today over the history of these warnings, one has the impression that something has now been lost of the sense of urgency, the hopes, and the excitement that initially inspired them so many years ago. One senses, even on the part of those who today most acutely perceive the problem and are inwardly most exercised about it, a certain discouragement, resignation, perhaps even despair, when it comes to the question of raising the subject again. The danger is so obvious. So much has already been said. What is to be gained by reiteration? What good would it now do? Look at the record.

Over all these years the competition in the development of nuclear weaponry has proceeded steadily, relentlessly, without the faintest regard for all these warning voices. We have gone on piling weapon upon weapon, missile upon missile, new levels of destructiveness upon old ones. We have done this helplessly, almost involuntarily, like the victims of some sort of hypnotism, like men in a dream, like lemmings heading for the sea, like the children of Hamlin marching blindly along behind their Pied Piper.

And the result is that today we have achieved, we and the Russians together, in the creation of these devices and their means of delivery, levels of redundancy of such grotesque dimensions as to defy rational understanding.

I say redundancy. I know of no better way to describe it. But actually, the word is too mild. It implies that there could be levels of these weapons that would not be redundant. Personally, I doubt that there could. I question whether these devices are really weapons at all. A true weapon is at best something with which you endeavor to affect the behavior of another society by influencing the minds, the calculations, the intentions, of the men that control it; it is not something with which you destroy indiscriminately the lives, the substance, the hopes, the culture, the civilization, of another people.

What a confession of intellectual poverty it would be—what a bankruptcy of intelligent statesmanship—if we had to admit that such blind, senseless acts of destruction were the best use we could make of what we have come to view as the leading elements of our military strength! To my mind, the nuclear bomb is the most useless weapon ever invented. It can be employed to no rational purpose. It is not even an effective defense against itself. It is only something with which, in a moment of petulance or panic, you commit such fearful acts of destruction as no sane person would ever wish to have upon his conscience.

There are those who will agree, with a sigh, to much of what I have said, but will point to the need for something called deterrence. This is, of course, a concept which attributes to others—to others who, like ourselves, were born of women, walk on two legs, and love their children, to human beings, in short—the most fiendish and inhuman of tendencies. But all right: accepting for the sake of argument the profound iniquity of these adversaries, no one could deny, I think, that the present Soviet and American arsenals, presenting over a million times the destructive power of the Hiroshima bomb, are simply fantastically redundant to the purpose in question.

If the same relative proportions were to be preserved, something well less than 70 per cent of these stocks would surely suffice for the most sanguine concepts of deterrence, whether as between the two nuclear superpowers or with relation to any of those other governments that have been so ill-advised as to enter upon the nuclear path. Whatever their suspicions of each other, there can be no excuse on the part of these two governments for holding, poised against each other and poised in a sense against the whole northern hemisphere, quantities of these weapons so vastly in excess of any rational and demonstrable requirements.

How have we got ourselves into this dangerous mess?

Let us not confuse the question by blaming it all on the Soviet adversaries. They have, of course, their share of the blame, and it began not later than their cavalier dismissal of the Baruch Plan so many years ago. They too have made their mistakes: and I should be the last to deny it. But we must remember that it has been we Americans who, at almost every step of the road, have taken the lead in the development of this sort of weaponry. It was we who first produced and tested such a device; we who were the first to raise its destructiveness to a new level with the hydrogen bomb; we who introduced the multiple warhead; we who declined every proposal for the renunciation of the principle of "first use"; and we alone, so help us God, who have used the weapon in anger against others, and against tens of thousands of helpless noncombatants at that.

I know that reasons were offered for some of these things. I know that others might have taken this sort of a lead, had we not done so. But let us not, in the face of this record, so lose ourselves in self-righteousness and hypocrisy as to forget our own measure of complicity in creating the situation we face today.

What is it then, if not our own will, and if not the supposed wickedness of our opponents, that has brought us to this pass?

The answer, I think, is clear. It is primarily the inner momentum, the independent compulsions that arise and take charge of great powers when they enter upon a competition with each other in the building up of major armaments of any sort.

This is nothing new. I am a diplomatic historian. I see this same phenomenon playing its fateful part in the relations among the great European powers as much as a century ago. I see this competitive buildup of armaments conceived initially as a means to an end but soon becoming an end itself. I see it taking possession of men's imagination and behavior, becoming a force in its own right, detaching itself from the political differences that initially inspired it, and then leading both parties, invariably and inexorably, to the war they no longer know how to avoid.

This is a species of fixation, brewed out of many components. There are fears, resentments, national pride, personal pride. There are misreadings of the adversary's intentions—sometimes even the refusal to consider them at all. There is the tendency of national communities to idealize themselves and to dehumanize the opponent. There is the blinkered, narrow vision of the professional military planner, and his tendency to make war inevitable by assuming its inevitability. Tossed together, these components form a powerful brew. They guide the fears and the ambitions of men. They seize the policies of government and whip them around like trees before the tempest.

Is it possible to break out of this charmed and vicious circle? It is sobering to recognize that no one, at least to my knowledge, has yet done so. But no one, for that matter, has ever been faced with such great catastrophe, such inalterable catastrophe, at the end of the line. Others, in earlier decades, could befuddle themselves with dreams or something called "victory." We, perhaps fortunately, are denied this seductive prospect. We have to break out of the circle. We have no other choice.

How are we to do it?

I must confess that I see no possibility of doing this by means of discussions along the lines of the negotiations that have been in progress, of and on, over this past decade, under the acronym of SALT. I regret, to be sure, that the most recent SALT agreement has not been ratified. I regret it, because if the benefits to be expected from that agreement were slight, its disadvantages were even slighter, and it had a symbolic value which should not have been so lightly sacrificed. But I have, I repeat, no illusion that negotiations on the SALT pattern—negotiations, that is, in which each side is obsessed with the chimera of relative advantage and strives only to retain a maximum of the weaponry for itself while putting its opponents to the maximum disadvantage—I have no illusion that such negotiations could ever be adequate to get us out of this hole. They are not a way of escape from the weapons race; they are an integral part of it.

Whoever does not understand that, when it comes to nuclear weapons, the whole concept of relative advantage is illusory—whoever does not understand that, when you are talking about absurd and preposterous quantities of overkill, the relative sizes of arsenals have no serious meaning—whoever does not understand that the danger lies not in the possibility that someone else might have more missiles and warheads than we do, but in the very existence of these unconscionable quantities of highly poisonous explosives, and their existence, above all, in hands as weak and shaky and undependable as those of ourselves or our adversaries or any other mere human beings; whoever does not understand these things is never going to guide us out of this increasingly dark and menacing forest of bewilderments into which we have all wandered.

I can see no way out of this dilemma other than by a bold and sweeping departure—a departure that would cut surgically through the exaggerated anxieties, the self-endangered nightmares, and the sophisticated mathematics of destruction in which we have all been entangled over these recent years, and that would permit us to move, with courage and decision, to the heart of the problem.

President Reagan recently said, and I think very wisely, that he would "negotiate as long as necessary to reduce the numbers of nuclear weapons to a point where neither side threatens the survival of the other." Now that is, of course, precisely the thought to which these present observations of mine are addressed. But I wonder whether the negotiations would really have to be at such great length. What I would like to see the President do, after due consultation with the Congress, would be to propose to the Soviet government an immediate across-the-board reduction by 50 percent of the nuclear arsenals now being maintained by the two superpowers—a reduction affecting in equal measure all forms of the weapon, strategic, medium range, and tactical, as well as all means of their delivery—all this to be implemented at once and without further wrangling among the experts, and to be subject to such national means of verification as now lie at the disposal of the two powers.

Whether the balance of reduction would be precisely even—whether it could be construed to favor statistically one side or the other—would not be the question. Once we start thinking that way, we would be back on the same old fateful track that has brought us where we are today. Whatever the precise results of such a reduction, there would still be plenty of overkill left—so much so that if this first operation were successful, I would then like to see a second one put in hand to rid us of at least two-thirds of what would be left.

Now I have, of course, no idea of the scientific aspects of such an operation; but I can imagine that serious problems might be presented by the task of removing, and disposing safely of, the radioactive contents of the many thousands of warheads that would have to be dismantled. Should this be the case, I would like to see the President couple his appeal for a 50 percent reduction with the proposal that there be established a joint Soviet-American scientific committee, under the chairmanship of a distinguished neutral figure, to study jointly and in all humility the problem not only of the safe disposal of these wastes but also the question of how they could be utilized in such a way as to make a positive contribution to human life, either in the two countries themselves or—perhaps preferably—elsewhere. In such a joint scientific venture, we might both atone for some of our past follies and lay the foundation for a more constructive relationship.

It will be said: this proposal, whatever its merits, deals with only a part of the problem. This is perfectly true. Behind it there would still lurk the serious political differences that now divide us from the Soviet Union. Behind it would still lie the problems recently treated, and still to be treated, in the SALT forum. Behind it would still lie the great question of the acceptability of war itself, any war, even a conventional one, as a means of solving problems among great industrial powers in this age of high technology. What has been suggested here would not prejudice the continued treatment of these questions just as today, in whatever forums and under whatever safeguards the two powers find necessary. The conflicts and arguments over these questions could all still proceed to the heart's content of all those who view them with such passionate commitment. The stakes would simply be smaller; and that would be a great relief to all of us.

What I have suggested is, of course, only a beginning. But a beginning has to be made somewhere; and if it has to be made, it is best that it should be made where the dangers are the greatest, and their necessity the least. If a step of this nature could be successfully taken, people might find the heart to tackle with greater confidence and determination the many problems that would still remain.

It will be argued that there would be risks involved. Possibly so. I do not see them. I do not deny the possibility. But if there are, so what? Is it possible to conceive of any dangers greater than those that lie at the end of the collision course on which we are now embarked? And, if not, why choose the greater—why choose, in fact, the greatest—of all risks, in the hopes of avoiding the lesser ones?

We are confronted here, my friends, with two courses. At the end of one lies hope—faint hope, if you will—uncertain hope, hope surrounded with dangers, if you insist. At the end of the other lies, so far as I am able to see, no hope at all. Can there be—in the light of our duty not just to ourselves (for we are all going to die sooner or later) but of our duty to our own kind, our duty to the continuity of the generations, our duty to the great experiment of civilized life on this rare and rich and marvelous planet—can there be, in the light of these claims on our loyalty, any question as to which course we should adopt?

In the final week of his life, Albert Einstein signed the last of the collective appeals against the development of nuclear weapons that he was ever to sign. He was dead before it appeared. But it was an appeal drafted, I gather, by Bertrand Russell. I had my differences with Russell at the time, as I do now in retrospect, but I would like to quote one sentence from the final paragraph of that statement, not only because it was the last one Einstein ever signed, but because it sums up, I think, all that I have to say on the subject. It reads as follows:

"We appeal, as human beings to human beings: Remember your humanity, and forget the rest."

APPENDIX C

THE NUCLEAR WEAPONS FREEZE CAMPAIGN —NAMES AND ADDRESSES

NATIONAL FREEZE CLEARINGHOUSE

Randall Kehler
Nuclear Weapons Freeze Campaign
4144 Lindell Boulevard
2nd Floor
St. Louis, Missouri 63108
(314) 533-1169

ALABAMA

Judy and Jack Cumbee
Rt. 3 Box 490
Tuskegee, Alabama 36083
(205) 727-6922

Judy Hand
Southern Organizing Committee
7715 A 7th Avenue South
Birmingham, Alabama 35206
(205) 838-1056

Roslyn Snider
American Friends Service Committee
Disarmament Program
560 Dauphine Street
Mobile, Alabama 36602
(205) 438-1603

ALASKA

John Havelock
2024 Esquire Drive
Anchorage, Alaska 99503
(907) 263-1810

ARIZONA

Edwina Vogan
Nuclear-Free State
1145 East 6th Street
Tucson, Arizona 85719
(602) 792-3517

Elaine G. Schwartz
Women's Party for Survival
5516 East Rosewood
Tucson, Arizona 85711

Michael Stock
Box 338 Lake Mary Road
Flagstaff, Arizona 86001
(602) 779-2665

CALIFORNIA

Harold Willens
Californians for a Bilateral Nuclear Weapons Freeze
7250 Franklin Avenue, Suite 101
Los Angeles, California 90046
(213) 876-5971

Pam Nichols
Northern California Nuclear Weapons Freeze
5480 College Avenue
Oakland, California 94618
(415) 652-5231

Anne Sutherland and Deborah Lorentz
Interfaith Center to Reverse the Arms Race
132 North Euclid Avenue
Pasadena, California 91101
(213) 449-9430

Maria Faer
Montclair Presbyterian Church
Freeze Task Force
270 Mountain Avenue
Piedmont, California 94611
(415) 653-6987

Jo Seidita
Sepulveda Unitarian Universalist
     Association
Freeze Ballot Initiative
9601 Corbin Avenue
Northridge, California 91324
(213) 886-4489

Chris Stowell
5102 Towle Court
San Diego, California 92105
(714) 282-4726

Gary Comer
Womens International League for
     Peace and Freedom
5725 North Maroa #218
Fresno, California 93704
(209) 358-4669

David Edinger
American Friends Service Com-
     mittee
980 North Fair Oaks Avenue
Pasadena, California 91103
(213) 791-1978

Chris Summerville
1075 Olive Drive, #7
Davis, California 95616

Shyrl Merrick, Steve Miller,
     Richard Archambault
San Jose Peace Center
520 South 10th Street
San Jose, California 95112
(408) 297-2299

Steve Ladd
War Resisters League
85 Carl Street
San Francisco, California 94117
(415) 731-1220

COLORADO

Helen Henry
Nuclear Weapons Facilities Task
     Force
American Friends Service Com-
     mittee
1660 Lafayette Street
Denver, Colorado 80218
(303) 832-4508

John D. Minear, Chairman
Interfaith Concerns and Action
     Committee
Box 387
Laporte, Colorado 80535
(303) 482-0151

Sister Mary Luke Tobin
Loretto Disarmament
2832 South Vrain Street
Denver, Colorado 80236
(303) 922-7141

Steve Ackerman, Ann Pryor
Poudre Nuclear Freeze Campaign
629 South Howes Street
Fort Collins, Colorado 80521
(303) 482-8487

Eric Killinger
Boulder County Campaign for a
     Weapons Freeze
P.O. Box 1992
Boulder, Colorado 80306
(303) 444-8921

Maxwell Aley
Aspen Peace Fellowship
720 East Hyman, Suite 301
Aspen, Colorado 81699
(303) 925-5953

Karla Koll
Pike's Peak Justice and Peace
     Commission
235 East Fountain Boulevard
Colorado Springs, Colorado
     80903
(303) 632-6189

CONNECTICUT

Marta Daniels
Connecticut Coalition for a Nu-
clear Arms Freeze
American Friends Service Com-
mittee
RD #1, Box 494
Voluntown, Connecticut 06384
(203) 376-4098

John Rolland
Health Professionals to Prevent
Nuclear War
165 Alden Avenue
New Haven, Connecticut 06515
(203) 387-7474

Paul Hodel
Peace Education and Action
Center
64 Edgewood Avenue
New Haven, Connecticut 06511
(203) 633-0120

Rox Speir
Nuclear Freeze Campaign
111 Whapley Street
Glastonbury, Connecticut 06033
(203) 633-0120

DELAWARE

Charles Zoeller
Pacem in Terris
American Friends Service Committee
1106 Adams Street
Wilmington, Delaware 19801
(302) 656-2721

David Nuttal
P.O. Box 91
Wilmington, Delaware 19899
(302) 654-3068

DISTRICT OF COLUMBIA

William J. Price
World Peacemakers
2852 Ontario Road, N.W.
Washington, D.C. 20009
(202) 265-7582

Edith Villastrigo
Women Strike for Peace
201 Massachusetts Avenue, N.E.
#102
Washington, D.C. 20002
(202) 546-7397

Kathy Rundy
D.C. Campaign for a Nuclear
Weapons Freeze
1169 Columbia Road, N.W.
#303
Washington, D.C. 20009
(202) 265-6316

Bob Alpern, Director
Government Relations Task Force
National Nuclear Weapons
Freeze Campaign
United Universalist Association
100 Maryland Avenue, N.E.
Washington, D.C. 20002
(202) 547-0254

Barry Israel
Clifford and Warnke
815 Connecticut Avenue, N.W.
Washington, D.C. 20006
(202) 828-4263

FLORIDA

Ethel Felts
Coalition for Arms Limitation
and Survival
Box 931
Miami, Florida 33133
(305) 856-6373

Bob Brister
American Friends Service Committee
Tampa Bay Program
130 19th Street, S.E.
St. Petersburg, Florida 33705
(813) 822-5522

Dave McLintock
Peace Fellowship of North
Florida
2257 Dellwood Avenue
Jacksonville, Florida 32204
(904) 354-7355

Ira Shorr
Tallahassee Peace Coalition
P.O. Box 20168
Tallahassee, Florida 32304
(904) 222-5845

Lillian Jaros
Coalition for Survival
5860 Midnight Pass Road, #20
Sarasota, Florida 33581
(813) 349-3983

Jean Beardsley
The Community Alliance for
     Peace Education
Route 3, Box 180F
Gainesville, Florida 32606
(904) 462-3201

GEORGIA

Chip Reynolds
American Friends Service Com-
     mittee
Regional Office
92 Piedmont Avenue, N.E.
Atlanta, Georgia 30303
(404) 586-0460

Mark Reeve
Clergy and Laity Concerned
222 East Lake Drive
Decatur, Georgia 30030
(404) 377-6516

HAWAII

Mike Cervice
General Delivery
Captain Cook, Hawaii 96704

IDAHO

Michael Jones
Snake River Alliance
Box 1731
Boise, Idaho 83701
(208) 345-4675

ILLINOIS

Bernice Bild
Illinois Nuclear Weapons Freeze
     Campaign

22 East Van Buren, 5th Floor
Chicago, Illinois 60605

Robert Cleland
Committee for a Nuclear Overkill
     Moratorium (NOMOR)
407 South Dearborn Street, #935
Chicago, Illinois 60605
 (312) 663-1246

Glenview Nuclear Weapons
     Freeze Campaign
1321 Sleepy Hollow Road
Glenview, Illinois 60025
(312) 724-8957

Rose Mary Meyer
Eighth Day Center for Justice
22 East Van Buren
Chicago, Illinois 60605
(312) 427-4351

Allen Howe
North Shore Peace Initiative
723 Seward
Evanston, Illinois 60202
(312) 475-3692

Mark Nation
Champagne/Urbana Peace Initia-
     tive
405 West Illinois
Urbana, Illinois 61801
(217) 328-5222

Sandy Berliant
Wilmette Nuclear Weapons
     Freeze Campaign
530 Knox
Wilmette, Illinois 60091
(312) 251-0830

Silvia Barge
Illinois Council of Churches
615 South 5th Street
Springfield, Illinois 62703
(217) 522-4415

Rich Hutchinson
Sylvia Johnson
American Friends Service Com-
     mittee
407 South Dearborn Street
Chicago, Illinois 60605
(312) 427-2533

Bob Stein
Clergy and Laity Concerned
542 South Dearborn
Chicago, Illinois 60605
(312) 922-8234

Rev. Richard Weston-Jones
2100 Half Day Road
Deerfield, Illinois 60015
(312) 234-2460

INDIANA

Brother William Mewes, CSC
Social Justice Commission
Holy Cross Brothers Center
Notre Dame, Indiana 46556
(219) 233-8273

Shirley Whiteside
Fellowship for Reconciliation
P.O. Box 25
North Manchester, Indiana 46962
(219) 982-4277

Don Nead
University Church
P.O. Box 3023, 320 North Street
West Lafayette, Indiana 47906
(317) 743-3861

Howard Alexander
Friends Coordinating Committee
    on Peace
Friends United Meeting
101 Quaker Hill Drive
Richmond, Indiana 47374
(317) 962-7573

Helen Kennedy
2750 Two World Drive
Columbus, Indiana 47201
(812) 379-2070

IOWA

Timothy Buttons
Iowa Freeze Campaign
4211 Grand Avenue
Des Moines, Iowa 50312
(515) 274-4851

Ron Nelson
Department of History
Northwestern College
Orange City, Iowa 51051
(712) 737-4821

Sally McMillan
Citizens for Peace
1825 Vogt
Burlington, Iowa 52601
(319) 753-1142, 754-4807

Jon Wacker
Freeze Iowa
RR 3, Box 229
Marion, Iowa 52302
(319) 377-2456

Marilyn Fenn
Freeze Iowa
2631 Knapp Street
Ames, Iowa 50010
(515) 292-4381

Rev. Charles Pullen
Prospect Hill Presbytery
Box 1405
Storm Lake, Iowa 50586
(712) 732-2097

Theresa Caluori
Catholic Peace Fellowship
1100 Carmel Drive
Dubuque, Iowa 52001
(319) 588-2351

Daniel Clark
Consortium of International
    Peace and Reconciliation
317 East 5th Street, #8
Des Moines, Iowa 50309
(515) 244-2253

KANSAS

Annabell Haupt
Kansans for Peace and Justice
1006 Amidon Street
Wichita, Kansas 67203
(316) 276-4197

Fred Loganhill
514 West 12th
Newton, Kansas 67114
(316) 284-2452

KENTUCKY

Pat McCullough
Council on Peacemaking and Religion
3940 Poplar Level Road
Louisville, Kentucky 40213
(502) 458-0269

Sister Jane Luttrell
4331 Hazelwood Avenue
Louisville, Kentucky 40215

Doris Firm
Central Kentucky Fellowship of
Reconciliation
812 Surrey Lane
Lexington, Kentucky 40503
(606) 278-2173

LOUISIANA

Joe McCarty
Lafayette Pax Christi
611 Taft Street
Lafayette, Louisiana 70503
(318) 233-5970

Herbert Rothschild
Center for Disarmament Education
P.O. Box 23790
Baton Rouge, Louisiana 70893
(504) 924-1519

MAINE

Deborah Hibbard
American Friends Service Committee
P.O. Box 7097
Lewiston, Maine 04240
(207) 772-0680, 784-1278

Pat Jones
Womens Party for Survival
Box 126
Kennebunk, Maine 04046
(207) 967-2375

Larry Dassinger
Maine Clergy and Laity Concerned
RFD 1
Newport, Maine 04953

MARYLAND

Barbara and Joseph Jensen
Fellowship of Reconciliation
One York Court
Baltimore, Maryland 21218
(301) 476-4611

Fran Donalan
Disarmament Program
American Friends Service Committee
317 East 25th Street
Baltimore, Maryland 21218
(301) 366-7200

Daniel L. Jerrems
Maryland Freeze Campaign
2702 Maryland Avenue
Baltimore, Maryland 21218
(301) 366-3758

Charles Maxwell
Cedar Lane Unitarians
Board of Social Concern
4510 Gretna Street
Bethesda, Maryland 20014
(301) 530-1683

Sarah Reese
Nuclear Arms Freeze Task Force
of Maryland
9601 Cedar Lane
Bethesda, Maryland 20814
(301) 593-4527

Dave Davis
1912 South Fountain Green Road
Bel Air, Maryland 21014
(301) 734-4148

MASSACHUSETTS

Pauline Bassett
Western Massachusetts Coalition
for a Nuclear Weapons
Freeze
Traprock Peace Center
Woolman Hill, Keets Road
Deerfield, Massachusetts 01342
(413) 773-5188

Frances Crowe
American Friends Service Committee
3 Langworthy Road
Northampton, Massachusetts
    01060
(413) 584-8975

Mark Niedergang, Melinda Fine
Institute for Defense and Disarmament Studies
251 Harvard Street
Brookline, Massachusetts 02146
(617) 734-4216

George Sommaripa
Council for a Nuclear Weapons
    Freeze
2161 Massachusetts Avenue
Cambridge, Massachusetts 02140
(617) 491-7809

Carla Johnston
Womens Action for Nuclear
    Disarmament
56 North Beacon Street
Watertown, Massachusetts 02172
(617) 923-9542

Reverend Edmund Brennan
Cape Cod Chapter
Fellowship of Reconciliation
32 Landings Drive, RR 3
Brewster, Massachusetts 02631
(617) 896-3106

Sally Gould
Needham Committee for a Nuclear Weapons Freeze
17 Coulton Park
Needham, Massachusetts 02192
(617) 444-0562

Gordon Harris
People for Peace
P.O. Box 537
Great Barrington, Massachusetts
    01230
(413) 229-3457

Abner Shimony
Wellesley Committee for a Nuclear Weapons Freeze
8 Dover Road
Wellesley, Massachusetts 02181
(617) 235-8485

Louise Bruyn
American Friends Service Committee
2161 Massachusetts Avenue
Cambridge, Massachusetts 02140
(617) 661-6130

Jane Parker
The Lower Cape Committee for
    a Nuclear Arms Freeze
Box 573
Truro, Massachusetts 02666
(617) 349-3358

Kathy Knight
Catholic Connection
27 Isabella Street
Boston, Massachusetts 02117
(617) 482-6295

Reverend Lloyd H. Dunham
The Second Congregational
    Church
Greenfield, Massachusetts 01301
(413) 774-4355

MICHIGAN

Interfaith Council for Peace
614 East Huron
Ann Arbor, Michigan 48104
(313) 663-1870

Debbie Heil, David Wysocki
Michigan Nuclear Weapons
    Freeze Campaign
P.O. Box 2257
Detroit, Michigan 48226
(313) 962-0416, 843-8171

Paul Dejong, Barbara Boylan
Institute for Global Education
25 Sheldon S.E., Suite 315
Grand Rapids, Michigan 49503
(616) 454-1642

Mary Curry
Peace and National Priorities
    Center of Oakland County
P.O. Box 5194
Orchard Lake, Michigan 48033
(313) 626-8396

Glen Rouse
Traverse Bay Area Nuclear
　　Weapons Freeze
P.O. Box 382
Traverse City, Michigan 49684
(616) 946-1638

MINNESOTA

Sister Kathleen Shields
Sisters of Saint Joseph of Caron-
　　dolet
1884 Randolph Avenue
St. Paul, Minnesota 55105
(612) 690-2481

Madge Michaels-Cyrus
People for Survival
1925 Nicollet Avenue, Suite 101
Minneapolis, Minnesota 55403
(612) 870-1501, 870-1540

Dianne Wanner
Clergy and Laity Concerned
122 West Franklin Street
Minneapolis, Minnesota 55404
(612) 817-8033

George E. Dizard
3925 London Road
Duluth, Minnesota 55804
(218) 525-3617

Cherie Lozier
Rt. 2, Box 184
Frontenac, Minnesota 55026

MISSISSIPPI

Carol Burnett
P.O. Box 87
Thomastown, Mississippi 39171
(601) 289-1839

MISSOURI

Bill Ramsey
American Friends Service Com-
　　mittee
438 North Skinker Boulevard
St. Louis, Missouri 63130
(314) 862-5770

Mary Alice Guilfoil, OSB
Peace House
3741 Forest Avenue
Kansas City, Missouri 64109

Francis Kenoyer
Loretto Disarmament
2544 Cherry Street
Kansas City, Missouri 64108
(816) 842-5170

Yvonne Logan
Womens International League for
　　Peace and Freedom
438 North Skinker Boulevard
St. Louis, Missouri 63130
(314) 449-5688

Randy Horn
Kansas City Nuclear Weapons
　　Freeze Coalition
629 West 39th Terrace
Kansas City, Missouri 64111
(816) 756-1904

MONTANA

Melissa Kwasny
Womens Party for Survival
Box 464
Basin, Montana 59631

Mike Kadas
Student Action Center
University Center 105
University of Montana
Missoula, Montana 59812
(406) 243-5897

NEBRASKA

Nebraskans for Peace
430 South 16th Street
Lincoln, Nebraska 68508
(402) 475-4620

Diane Schuette
Omaha Coalition to Freeze the
　　Arms Race
2104 Davenport
Omaha, Nebraska 68102
(402) 345-0539

NEVADA

Rosemary Lynch
Sagebrush Alliance
704 West McWilliams Avenue
Las Vegas, Nevada 89106
(702) 647-3610

NEW HAMPSHIRE

Arnie Alpert
American Friends Service Com-
mittee
Box 1081, 77 North Main
Concord, New Hampshire 03301
(603) 224-2407

Harriet V. Allen
Coalition for Peoples Rights and
Survival
P.O. Box 1032
Dover, New Hampshire 03820
(603) 749-4076

NEW JERSEY

Dorothy Eldridge
New Jersey SANE
324 Bloomfield Avenue
Montclair, New Jersey 07042
(201) 744-3263

Rev. Bob Moore
Coalition for Nuclear Disarmament
20 Nassau Street, Room 501
Princeton, New Jersey 08540
(609) 924-5022

Frank Askin
Coalition for Human Priorities
23 Beaumont Terrace
West Orange, New Jersey 07052
(201) 731-2355

NEW MEXICO

Dorie Bunting
New Mexico Peace Conversion
5021 Guadalupe Trail, N.W.
Albuquerque, New Mexico 87107
(505) 334-1140

Dianne Andrews
New Mexicans for a Bilateral
Nuclear Weapons Freeze
2425 Alamo Avenue S.E.
Albuquerque, New Mexico
87106
(505) 255-0381

Bruce Berlin
Santa Fe Peace Coalition
128 Lugar de Oro
Santa Fe, New Mexico 85701

NEW YORK

Patsy Leake
American Friends Service Committee
New Manhattan Project
15 Rutherford Place
New York, New York 10003
(212) 598-0971

James Mang
Western New York Peace Center
440 Leroy Avenue
Buffalo, New York 14215
(716) 835-4073

Rod Morris
Peace Associates
Box 386
Oxford, New York 13830
(607) 843-9382

Reverend James Van Hoeven,
Patricia Beetle
Nuclear Weapons Freeze Campaign
727 Madison Avenue
Albany, New York 12208
(518) 477-4004, 466-4449

Alice Daly
Nuclear Weapons Freeze Campaign Suffolk
12 Maple Street
Port Jefferson Station, New York
11776
(516) 928-5555

Ruth Yarrow
Tompkins County Freeze Campaign
407 Hancock
Ithaca, New York 14850
(607) 272-4943

Virden Seybold
American Friends Service Committee
Upper New York State Area
821 Euclid Avenue
Syracuse, New York 13210
(315) 475-4822

Robert Staley-Mays
Peace and Justice Education Center
713 Monroe Avenue
Rochester, New York 14607
(716) 244-7191

Cora Weiss
The Riverside Church Disarmament Program
490 Riverside Drive
New York, New York 10027
(212) 222-5900

Rev. Kenneth R. Brown
North Shore Unitarian Church
Plandome Road
Westgate Boulevard
Plandome, New York 10030
(516) 627-6560

Marty Bartlett
Central New York Freeze Campaign
103 Rita Drive
North Syracuse, New York 13212
(315) 458-6266

NORTH CAROLINA

Mark Legerton/Donna Chavis
Robeson County Clergy and Laity Concerned
P.O. Box 9
Pembroke, North Carolina 28372
(919) 521-3269

Anne Welsh
American Friends Service Committee
P.O. Box 2234
High Point North Carolina 27261
(919) 882-0109

Steve Summerford
War Resisters League/Southeast
604 West Chapel Hill Street
Durham, North Carolina 27701
(919) 682-6374

Ellen Krebs and Rev. H. Lull
Franklin Peace Fellowship
Rt. 3, Box 116A
Franklin, North Carolina 28734

John Stevens
University of North Carolina
University Heights
Asheville, North Carolina 28814
(704) 258-6600

Ron Shackelford
Coastal Alliance for a Safe Environment
105 Kenwood Avenue
Wilmington, North Carolina 28405
(919) 762-8530

NORTH DAKOTA

Louise Pare, Paula Youndale
North Dakota Peace Network
Box 782
Mandan, North Dakota 58554
(701) 663-6522, 222-2918

OHIO

Saran Kirschenbaum
Reverse the Arms Race Federation of Ohio
Ohio Nuclear Weapons Freeze at the Holy Family Peace Center
584 West Broad
Columbus, Ohio 43215
(614) 221-3741

John Looney
Columbus Area Nuclear Weapons
    Freeze Campaign
c/o American Friends Services
    Committee
475 West Market Street
Akron, Ohio 44303
(216) 335-1593, 253-7151

Peter Shidemantle
Swords into Plowshares
14321 Detroit Avenue
Lakewood, Ohio 44107
(216) 221-7264

John Rider
Reverse the Arms Race Feder-
    ation of Ohio
3800 Bridge Avenue
Cleveland, Ohio 44113
(216) 281-2600

OKLAHOMA

Hugh Tribbey
Enid Arms Reduction Task Force
1802 East Park
Enid, Oklahoma 73701

Jim Bowers
Oklahoma Peace Center
1829 Gatewood
Oklahoma City, Oklahoma 73106
(405) 524-1493, 632-7574

Rex Friend
2937 Northwest 17th Street
Oklahoma City, Oklahoma 73107
(405) 949-1928

OREGON

Peter Bergel
Citizens Action for Lasting Se-
    curity
Box 12763
Salem, Oregon 97303
(503) 371-8002, 364-9457

Steven Pettengill
Citizens Action for Lasting Se-
    curity
P.O. Box 12229
Portland, Oregon 97212
(503) 243-2257

Hal Darst
Citizens Action for Lasting Se-
    curity
454 Willamette Street
Eugene, Oregon 97401
(503) 343-8548

Carl Eggers
Citizens Action for Lasting Se-
    curity
221 Granite Street
Ashland, Oregon 97520
(503) 482-9787

Karen Steingart
Physicians for Social Responsi-
    bility
P.O. Box 1472
Portland, Oregon 97214
(503) 245-5154, 239-8556

Nora Hallet
Oregon Fellowship of Reconcilia-
    tion
1838 S.W. Jefferson
Portland, Oregon 97201
(503) 222-7293

PENNSYLVANIA

Billy Grassie
Pennsylvania Campaign for a Nu-
    clear Weapons Freeze
1515 Cherry Street
Philadelphia, Pennsylvania 19102
(215) 241-7230

Marlene Bertke, OSB
Pax Center, 345 East 9th Street
Erie, Pennsylvania 16503

Juli Loesch
Prolifers for Survival
252 East 9th Street
Erie, Pennsylvania 16505
(814) 456-1791

Nancy Strong
Bucks County Womens Interna-
    tional League for Peace and
    Freedom
120 South Chancellor Street
Newtown, Pennsylvania 18940

Bob Ellenberg
Wayne Citizens for a Nuclear
    Weapons Freeze
950 Maple Avenue
Homesdale, Pennsylvania 18431
(717) 253-4051

RHODE ISLAND

Carol Bragg
American Friends Service Com-
    mittee
2 Stimson Avenue
Providence, Rhode Island 02906
(401) 751-4488

SOUTH DAKOTA

Tim Langley
South Dakota Peace and Justice
    Center
Box 405
Watertown, South Dakota 57201
(605) 882-2822

TENNESSEE

Joceline Lemaire
Nashville Clergy and Laity Con-
    cerned
P.O. Box 90557
Nashville, Tennessee 37209
(615) 292-7607

Sam H. Franklin, Jr.
Bread for the World
513 Court Street
Maryville, Tennessee 37801
(615) 984-3908

Rev. Thomas Kirchberg
3867 Summer Avenue
Memphis, Tennessee 38122

Jason Lee
1688 Carruthers Place #7
Memphis, Tennessee 38112
(901) 278-3556

Barbara Mann
Tennessee Nuclear Weapons
    Freeze Campaign
3730 Westport Drive
Nashville, Tennessee 37218
(615) 876-3114

TEXAS

Mary Peter Bruce
Loretto Disarmament Committee
1300 Hardaway Street
El Paso, Texas 79903
(915) 566-1628

Northwest Texas Clergy and
    Laity Concerned
3500 South Bowie Street
Amarillo, Texas 79109

Mr. and Ms. William C. Hardt
Ecumenical Peace Force
4907 Caris Street
Houston, Texas 77091
(713) 688-3803

Roxanne Elder
Texas Mobilization for Survival
1022 West 6th Street
Austin, Texas 78703
(512) 474-2399

Ann Wharton
Citizens Anti-Nuclear Information
    Team (CAN-IT)
1401 Harold Street
Houston, Texas 77006
(713) 528-0397

Deane Orr
Citizens for Education on Nu-
    clear Arms
2229 Winton Terrace West
Fort Worth, Texas 76109
(817) 926-3827

Tony Switzer
Nuclear Weapons Freeze Cam-
    paign
Box 4413
Austin, Texas 78765
(512) 476-3294

UTAH

Janet Gordon
Citizens Call in Utah
126 South 1400 West
Cedar City, Utah 84720
(801) 586-6674

Stan Holmes
MX Information Center
232½ University Street
Salt Lake City, Utah 84102
(801) 581-9027

VERMONT

David McCauley
American Friends Service Committee
RD 1
Putney, Vermont 05346
(802) 387-5732

Rev. Howard Stearns
Vermont Ecumenical Peace Committee
P.O. Box 593
Burlington, Vermont 05402
(802) 658-2540

The Norwich Center
Main Street
Norwich, Vermont 05055
(802) 649-1000

VIRGINIA

Norman Jimerson
Plowshare Peace Center
Box 1623
Roanoke, Virginia 24008
(703) 985-0808

Steve Hodges
Peace Education Center
14 North Laurel Street
Richmond, Virginia 23220
(804) 358-1958

Phyllis Conklin
Womens International League for Peace and Freedom
Richmond Nuclear Freeze Campaign
8429 Ben Nevis Drive
Bel Air, Virginia 23235
(804) 272-1851

Nan Rodney
Virginia Nuclear Weapons Freeze Campaign

6718 Rolling Road
Springfield, Virginia 22162
(703) 451-5657

Scott Moore
Nuclear Weapons Freeze Campaign
947 Rockcreek Road
Charlottesville, Virginia 22903
(804) 295-0033

WASHINGTON

Mark Plunkett
Nuclear Weapons Freeze Campaign
4534½ University Way N.E.
Seattle, Washington 98105

Ruth Hood
Armistice
2524 16th Street South
Seattle, Washington 98102
(206) 324-1489

Nick Kassenbaum
224 East Sharp Avenue
Spokane, Washington 99202

Alice Litton
Nuclear Weapons Freeze Campaign
520 17th Street
Bellingham, Washington 98225
(206) 676-8951

WEST VIRGINIA

Tom Hougham
Allies Waged Against a Radioactive Environment (AWARE)
4030 Clark Graham Road
Huntington, West Virginia 25710
(304) 529-3643

Mike Kelly
Box 247
Charleston, West Virginia 25321
(304) 342-2395

WISCONSIN

Michael Trokan
Justice and Peace Center
1016 North 9th Street
Milwaukee, Wisconsin 53233
(414) 272-0272

Dick Bruefehoff
Ecumenical Partnership for Peace
    and Justice
Route 2, Box 161
Turtle Lake, Wisconsin 54889
(715) 268-2816

Trudy Carlson
Wisconsin Nuclear Weapons
    Freeze Campaign
315 West Gorham Street

Madison, Wisconsin 53703
(608) 256-4146

Lynette Biesamy
Citizens Against Nuclear Arms
Route 1
Cochrane, Wisconsin 54722
(608) 626-3331

WYOMING

Mignon and John Hill
264 North 9th Street
Laramie, Wyoming 82070
(307) 742-2259

Francis Russell, SCL
720 West 25th Street
Cheyenne, Wyoming 82001

Appendix D

MEMBERS OF CONGRESS

ALABAMA
Senate
Howell Heflin (Democrat)
Jeremiah Denton (Republican)
House of Representatives
Jack Edwards (Republican) (First District)
William L. Dickinson (Republican) (Second District)
Bill Nichols (Democrat) (Third District)
Tom Bevill (Democrat) (Fourth District)
Ronnie G. Flippo (Democrat) (Fifth District)
Albert Lee Smith, Jr. (Republican) (Sixth District)
Richard C. Shelby (Democrat) (Seventh District)

ALASKA
Senate
Ted Stevens (Republican)
Frank H. Murkowski (Republican)
House of Representatives
Don Young (Republican)

ARIZONA
Senate
Barry Goldwater (Republican)
Dennis DeConcini (Democrat)
House of Representatives
John J. Rhodes (Republican) (First District)
Morris K. Udall (Democrat) (Second District)
Bob Stump (Democrat) (Third District)
Eldon Rudd (Republican) (Fourth District)

ARKANSAS
Senate
Dale Bumpers (Democrat)
David Pryor (Democrat)
House of Representatives
Bill Alexander (Democrat) (First District)
Ed Bethune (Republican) (Second District)

John Paul Hammerschmidt (Republican) (Third District)
Beryl F. Anthony, Jr. (Democrat) (Fourth District)

CALIFORNIA
Senate
Alan Cranston (Democrat)
S. I. Hayakawa (Republican)
House of Representatives
Eugene A. Chappie (Republican) (First District)
Don H. Clausen (Republican) (Second District)
Robert T. Matsui (Democrat) (Third District)
Vic Fazio (Democrat) (Fourth District)
John L. Burton (Democrat) (Fifth District)
Phillip Burton (Democrat) (Sixth District)
George Miller (Democrat) (Seventh District)
Ronald V. Dellums (Democrat) (Eighth District)
Fortney H. (Pete) Stark (Democrat) (Ninth District)
Don Edwards (Democrat) (Tenth District)
Tom Lantos (Democrat) (Eleventh District)
Paul N. McCloskey, Jr. (Republican) (Twelfth District)
Norman Y. Mineta (Democrat) (Thirteenth District)
Norman D. Shumway (Republican) (Fourteenth District)
Tony Coelho (Democrat) (Fifteenth District)
Leon E. Panetta (Democrat) (Sixteenth District)
Charles (Chip) Pashayan, Jr. (Republican) (Seventeenth District)
William M. Thomas (Republican) (Eighteenth District)
Robert J. Lagomarsino (Republican) (Nineteenth District)
Barry M. Goldwater, Jr. (Republican) (Twentieth District)
Bobbi Fiedler (Republican) (Twenty-First District)
Carlos J. Moorhead (Republican) (Twenty-Second District)
Anthony C. Beilenson (Democrat) (Twenty-Third District)
Henry A. Waxman (Democrat) (Twenty-Fourth District)
Edward R. Roybal (Democrat) (Twenty-Fifth District)
John Rousselot (Republican) (Twenty-Sixth District)
Robert K. Dornan (Republican) (Twenty-Seventh District)
Julian C. Dixon (Democrat) (Twenty-Eighth District)
Augustus F. Hawkins (Democrat) (Twenty-Ninth District)
(Thirtieth District - Vacancy)
Mervyn M. Dymally (Democrat) (Thirty-First District)
Glenn M. Anderson (Democrat) (Thirty-Second District)
Wayne Grisham (Republican) (Thirty-Third District)
Daniel E. (Dan) Lungren (Republican) (Thirty-Fourth District)
David Dreier (Republican) (Thirty-Fifth District)
George E. Brown, Jr. (Democrat) (Thirty-Sixth District)
Jerry Lewis (Republican) (Thirty-Seventh District)
Jerry M. Patterson (Democrat) (Thirty-Eighth District)
William E. Dannemeyer (Republican) (Thirty-Ninth District)
Robert E. Badham (Republican) (Fortieth District)
Bill Lowery (Republican) (Forty-First District)
Duncan L. Hunter (Republican) (Forty-Second District)
Clair W. Burgener (Republican) (Forty-Third District)

COLORADO
Senate
Gary W. Hart (Democrat)
William L. Armstrong (Republican)
House of Representatives
Patricia Schroeder (Democrat) (First District)
Timothy E. Wirth (Democrat) (Second District)
Ray Kogovsek (Democrat) (Third District)
Hank Brown (Republican) (Fourth District)
Ken Kramer (Republican) (Fifth District)

CONNECTICUT
Senate
Lowell P. Weicker, Jr. (Republican)
Christopher J. Dodd (Democrat)
House of Representatives
Barbara Kennelly (Democrat) (First District)
Samuel Gejdenson (Democrat) (Second District)
Lawrence J. DeNardis (Republican) (Third District)
Stewart B. McKinney (Republican) (Fourth District)
William R. Ratchford (Democrat) (Fifth District)
Anthony Toby Moffett (Democrat) (Sixth District)

DELAWARE
Senate
William V. Roth, Jr. (Republican)
Joseph R. Biden, Jr. (Democrat)
House of Representatives
Thomas B. Evans, Jr. (Republican)

FLORIDA
Senate
Lawton Chiles (Democrat)
Paula Hawkins (Republican)
House of Representatives
Earl Dewitt Hutto (Democrat) (First District)
Don Fuqua (Democrat) (Second District)
Charles E. Bennett (Democrat) (Third District)
Bill Chappell, Jr. (Democrat) (Fourth District)
Bill McCollum (Republican) (Fifth District)
C. W. Bill Young (Republican) (Sixth District)
Sam Gibbons (Democrat) (Seventh District)
Andy Ireland (Democrat) (Eighth District)
Bill Nelson (Democrat) (Ninth District)
L. A. (Skip) Bafalis (Republican) (Tenth District)
Dan Mica (Democrat) (Eleventh District)
E. Clay Shaw, Jr. (Republican) (Twelfth District)
William Lehman (Democrat) (Thirteenth District)
Claude Pepper (Democrat) (Fourteenth District)
Dante B. Fascell Democrat) (Fifteenth District)

GEORGIA

Senate

Sam Nunn (Democrat)

Mack Mattingly (Republican)

House of Representatives

Bo Ginn (Democrat) (First District)

Charles F. Hatcher (Democrat) (Second District)

Jack Brinkley (Democrat) (Third District)

Elliott H. Levitas (Democrat) (Fourth District)

Wyche Fowler, Jr. (Democrat) (Fifth District)

Newt Gingrich (Republican) (Sixth District)

Larry P. McDonald (Democrat) (Seventh District)

Billy Lee Evans (Democrat) (Eighth District)

Ed Jenkins (Democrat) (Ninth District)

Doug Barnard, Jr. (Democrat) (Tenth District)

HAWAII

Senate

Daniel K. Inouye (Democrat)

Spark M. Matsunaga (Democrat)

House of Representatives

Cecil Heftel (Democrat) (First District)

Daniel K. Akaka (Democrat) (Second District)

IDAHO

Senate

James A. McClure (Republican)

Steven D. Symms (Republican)

House of Representatives

Larry Craig (Republican) (First District)

George Hansen (Republican) (Second District)

ILLINOIS

Senate

Charles H. Percy (Republican)

Alan J. Dixon (Democrat)

House of Representatives

Harold Washington (Democrat) (First District)

Gus Savage (Democrat) (Second District)

Martin A. (Marty) Russo (Democrat) (Third District)

Edward J. Derwinski (Republican) (Fourth District)

John G. Fary (Democrat) (Fifth District)

Henry J. Hyde (Republican) (Sixth District)

Cardiss Collins (Democrat) (Seventh District)

Dan Rostenkowski (Democrat) (Eighth District)

Sidney R. Yates (Democrat) (Ninth District)

John E. Porter (Republican) (Tenth District)

Frank Annunzio (Democrat) (Eleventh District)

Philip M. Crane (Republican) (Twelfth District)

Robert McClory (Republican) (Thirteenth District)

John N. Erlenborn (Republican) (Fourteenth District)

Tom Corcoran (Republican) (Fifteenth District)
Lynn M. Martin (Republican) (Sixteenth District)
George M. O'Brien (Republican) (Seventeenth District)
Robert M. Michel (Republican) (Eighteenth District)
Tom Railsback (Republican) (Nineteenth District)
Paul Findley (Republican) (Twentieth District)
Edward R. Madigan (Republican) (Twenty-First District)
Daniel B. Crane (Republican) (Twenty-Second District)
Melvin Price (Democrat) (Twenty-Third District)
Paul Simon (Democrat) (Twenty-Fourth District)

INDIANA

Senate
Richard G. Lugar (Republican)
Dan Quayle (Republican)
House of Representatives
Adam Benjamin, Jr. (Democrat) (First District)
Floyd J. Fithian (Democrat) (Second District)
John P. Hiler (Republican) (Third District)
Daniel R. Coats (Republican) (Fourth District)
Elwood R. Hillis (Republican) (Fifth District)
David W. Evans (Democrat) (Sixth District)
John T. Myers (Republican) (Seventh District)
H. Joel Deckard (Republican) (Eighth District)
Lee H. Hamilton, Jr. (Democrat) (Ninth District)
Philip R. Sharp (Democrat) (Tenth District)
Andrew Jacobs, Jr. (Democrat) (Eleventh District)

IOWA

Senate
Roger W. Jepsen (Republican)
Charles E. Grassley (Republican)
House of Representatives
James A. S. (Jim) Leach (Republican) (First District)
Thomas J. Tauke (Republican) (Second District)
Cooper Evans (Republican) (Third District)
Neal Smith (Democrat) (Fourth District)
Tom Harkin (Democrat) (Fifth District)
Berkley Bedell (Democrat) (Sixth District)

KANSAS

Senate
Robert Dole (Republican)
Nancy Landon Kassebaum (Republican)
House of Representatives
Pat Roberts (Republican) (First District)
Jim Jeffries (Republican) (Second District)
Larry Winn, Jr. (Republican) (Third District)
Dan Glickman (Democrat) (Fourth District)
Robert (Bob) Whittaker (Republican) (Fifth District)

KENTUCKY
Senate
Walter D. (Dee) Huddleston (Democrat)
Wendell H. Ford (Democrat)
House of Representatives
Carroll Hubbard, Jr. (Democrat) (First District)
William H. Natcher (Democrat) (Second District)
Ramano L. Mazzoli (Democrat) (Third District)
Gene Snyder (Republican) (Fourth District)
Harold Rogers (Republican) (Fifth District)
Larry J. Hopkins (Republican) (Sixth District)
Carl D. Perkins (Democrat) (Seventh District)

LOUISIANA
Senate
Russell B. Long (Democrat)
J. Bennett Johnston, Jr. (Democrat)
House of Representatives
Robert L. (Bob) Livingston (Republican) (First District)
Lindy (Mrs. Hale) Boggs (Democrat) (Second District)
Wilbert J. (Billy) Tauzin (Democrat) (Third District)
Buddy Roemer (Democrat) (Fourth District)
Jerry Huckaby (Democrat) (Fifth District)
W. Henson Moore (Republican) (Sixth District)
John B. Breaux (Democrat) (Seventh District)
Gillis W. Long (Democrat) (Eighth District)

MAINE
Senate
William S. Cohen (Republican)
George J. Mitchell (Democrat)
House of Representatives
David F. Emery (Republican) (First District)
Olympia J. Snowe (Republican) (Second District)

MARYLAND
Senate
Charles McC. Mathias, Jr. (Republican)
Paul S. Sarbanes (Democrat)
House of Representatives
Roy Dyson (Democrat) (First District)
Clarence D. Long (Democrat) (Second District)
Barbara A. Mikulski (Democrat) (Third District)
Marjorie S. Holt (Republican) (Fourth District)
Steny H. Hoyer (Democrat) (Fifth District)
Beverly B. Byron (Democrat) (Sixth District)
Parren J. Mitchell (Democrat) (Seventh District)
Michael D. Barnes (Democrat) (Eighth District)

MASSACHUSETTS
Senate
Edward M. Kennedy (Democrat)
Paul E. Tsongas (Democrat)
House of Representatives
Silvio O. Conte (Republican) (First District)
Edward P. Boland (Democrat) (Second District)
Joseph D. Early (Democrat) (Third District)
Barney Frank (Democrat) (Fourth District)
James M. Shannon (Democrat) (Fifth District)
Nicholas Mavroules (Democrat) (Sixth District)
Edward J. Markey (Democrat) (Seventh District)
Thomas P. (Tip) O'Neill, Jr. (Democrat) (Eighth District)
John Joseph (Joe) Moakley (Democrat) (Ninth District)
Margaret M. Heckler (Republican) (Tenth District)
Brian J. Donnelly (Democrat) (Eleventh District)
Gerry E. Studds (Democrat) (Twelfth District)

MICHIGAN
Senate
Donald W. Riegle, Jr. (Democrat)
Carl Levin (Democrat)
House of Representatives
John Conyers, Jr. (Democrat) (First District)
Carl D. Pursell (Republican) (Second District)
Howard Wolpe (Democrat) (Third District)
Mark Siljander (Republican) (Fourth District)
Harold S. Sawyer (Republican) (Fifth District)
Jim Dunn (Republican) (Sixth District)
Dale E. Kildee (Democrat) (Seventh District)
Bob Traxler (Democrat) (Eighth District)
Guy Vander Jagt (Republican) (Ninth District)
Donald Joseph (Don) Albosta (Democrat) (Tenth District)
Robert W. (Bob) Davis (Republican) (Eleventh District)
David E. Bonior (Democrat) (Twelfth District)
George W. Crockett, Jr. (Democrat) (Thirteenth District)
Dennis Hertel (Democrat) (Fourteenth District)
William D. Ford (Democrat) (Fifteenth District)
John D. Dingell (Democrat) (Sixteenth District)
William M. Brodhead (Democrat) (Seventeenth District)
James J. (Jim) Blanchard (Democrat) (Eighteenth District)
William S. Broomfield (Republican) (Nineteenth District)

MINNESOTA
Senate
David Durenberger (Independent Republican)
Rudy Boschwitz (Independent Republican)
House of Representatives
Arlen Erdahl (Independent Republican) (First District)
Tom Hagedorn (Independent Republican) (Second District)
Bill Frenzel (Independent Republican) (Third District)

Bruce F. Vento (Democratic-Farmer-Labor) (Fourth District)
Martin Olav Sabo (Democratic-Farmer-Labor) (Fifth District)
Vin Weber (Independent Republican) (Sixth District)
Arlan Stangeland (Independent Republican) (Seventh District)
James L. Oberstar (Democratic-Farmer-Labor) (Eighth District)

MISSISSIPPI
Senate
John C. Stennis (Democrat)
Thad Cochran (Republican)
House of Representatives
Jamie L. Whitten (Democrat) (First District)
David R. Bowen (Democrat) (Second District)
G. V. (Sonny) Montgomery (Democratic) (Third District)
Wayne Dowdy (Democrat) (Fourth District)
Trent Lott (Republican) (Fifth District)

MISSOURI
Senate
Thomas F. Eagleton (Democrat)
John C. Danforth (Republican)
House of Representatives
William (Bill) Clay (Democrat) (First District)
Robert A. Young (Democrat) (Second District)
Richard A. Gephardt (Democrat) (Third District)
Ike Skelton (Democrat) (Fourth District)
Richard Bolling (Democrat) (Fifth District)
E. Thomas (Tom) Coleman (Republican) (Sixth District)
Gene Taylor (Republican) (Seventh District)
Wendell Bailey (Republican) (Eighth District)
Harold L. Volkmer (Democrat) (Ninth District)
Bill Emerson (Republican) (Tenth District)

MONTANA
Senate
John Melcher (Democrat)
Max Baucus (Democrat)
House of Representatives
Pat Williams (Democrat) (First District)
Ron Marlenee (Republican) (Second District)

NEBRASKA
Senate
Edward Zorinsky (Democrat)
James Exon (Democrat)
House of Representatives
Douglas (Doug) K. Bereuter (Republican) (First District)
Harold J. Daub (Republican) (Second District)
Virginia Smith (Republican) (Third District)

NEVADA
Senate
Howard W. Cannon (Democrat)
Paul Laxalt (Republican)
House of Representatives
Jim Santini (Democrat)

NEW HAMPSHIRE
Senate
Gordon J. Humphrey (Republican)
Warren Rudman (Republican)
House of Representatives
Norman E. D'Amours (Democrat) (First District)
Judd Gregg (Republican) (Second District)

NEW JERSEY
Senate
Bill Bradley (Democrat)
Nicholas F. Bradey (Republican)
House of Representatives
James J. Florio (Democrat) (First District)
William J. Hughes (Democrat) (Second District)
James J. Howard (Democrat) (Third District)
Christopher H. Smith (Republican) (Fourth District)
Millicent Fenwick (Republican) (Fifth District)
Edwin B. Forsythe (Republican) (Sixth District)
Margaret S. (Marge) Roukema (Republican) (Seventh District)
Robert A. Roe (Democrat) (Eighth District)
Harold C. Hollenbeck (Republican) (Ninth District)
Peter W. Rodino, Jr. (Democrat) (Tenth District)
Joseph G. Minish (Democrat) (Eleventh District)
Matthew J. Rinaldo (Republican) (Twelfth District)
James A. (Jim) Courter (Republican) (Thirteenth District)
Frank J. Guarini (Democrat) (Fourteenth District)
Bernard J. Dwyer (Democrat) (Fifteenth District)

NEW MEXICO
Senate
Pete V. Domenici (Republican)
Harrison H. (Jack) Schmitt (Republican)
House of Representatives
Manuel Lujan, Jr. (Republican) (First District)
Joseph R. Skeen (Republican) (Second District)

NEW YORK
Senate
Daniel Patrick Moynihan (Democrat)
Alfonse M. D'Amato (Republican)
House of Representatives
William Carney (Republican) (First District)
Thomas J. Downey (Democrat) (Second District)

Gregory W. Carman (Republican) (Third District)
Norman F. Lent (Republican) (Fourth District)
Raymond J. McGrath (Republican) (Fifth District)
John Le Boutillier (Republican) (Sixth District)
Joseph P. Addabbo (Democrat) (Seventh District)
Benjamin S. Rosenthal (Democrat) (Eighth District)
Geraldine A. Ferraro (Democrat) (Ninth District)
Mario Biaggi (Democrat) (Tenth District)
James H. Scheuer (Democrat) (Eleventh District)
Shirley Chisholm (Democrat) (Twelfth District)
Stephen J. Solarz (Democrat) (Thirteenth District)
Frederick W. Richmond (Democrat) (Fourteenth District)
Leo C. Zeferetti (Democrat) (Fifteenth District)
Charles E. Schumer (Democrat) (Sixteenth District)
Guy V. Molinari (Republican) (Seventeenth District)
S. William (Bill) Green (Republican) (Eighteenth District)
Charles B. Rangel (Democrat) (Nineteenth District)
Theodore S. (Ted) Weiss (Democrat) (Twentieth District)
Robert Garcia (Democrat) (Twenty-First District)
Jonathan B. Bingham (Democrat) (Twenty-Second District)
Peter A. Peyser (Democrat) (Twenty-Third District)
Richard L. Ottinger (Democrat) (Twenty-Fourth District)
Hamilton Fish, Jr. (Republican) (Twenty-Fifth District)
Benjamin A. Gilman (Republican) (Twenty-Sixth District)
Matthew F. McHugh (Democrat) (Twenty-Seventh District)
Samuel S. Stratton (Democrat) (Twenty-Eighth District)
Gerald B. H. Solomon (Republican) (Twenty-Ninth District)
David O'B. Martin (Republican) (Thirtieth District)
Donald J. Mitchell (Republican) (Thirty-First District)
George C. Wortley (Republican) (Thirty-Second District)
Gary A. Lee (Republican) (Thirty-Third District)
Frank Horton (Republican) (Thirty-Fourth District)
Barber B. Conable, Jr. (Republican) (Thirty-Fifth District)
John J. LaFalce (Democrat) (Thirty-Sixth District)
Henry J. Nowak (Democrat) (Thirty-Seventh District)
Jack F. Kemp (Republican) (Thirty-Eighth District)
Stanley N. Lundine (Democrat) (Thirty-Ninth District)

NORTH CAROLINA
Senate
Jesse A. Helms (Republican)
John P. East (Republican)
House of Representatives
Walter B. Jones (Democrat) (First District)
L. H. Fountain (Democrat) (Second District)
Charles O. Whitley (Democrat) (Third District)
Ike F. Andrews (Democrat) (Fourth District)
Stephen L. Neal (Democrat) (Fifth District)
Eugene Johnston (Republican) (Sixth District)
Charles G. (Charlie) Rose (Democrat) (Seventh District)
W. G. (Bill) Hefner (Democrat) (Eighth District)
James G. Martin (Republican) (Ninth District)

James T. Broyhill (Republican) (Tenth District)
William M. Hendon (Republican) (Eleventh District)

NORTH DAKOTA
Senate
Quentin N. Burdick (Democrat)
Mark Andrews (Republican)
House of Representatives
Byron L. Dorgan (Democrat)

OHIO
Senate
John H. Glenn, Jr. (Democrat)
Howard M. Metzenbaum (Democrat)
House of Representatives
Willis D. Gradison, Jr. (Republican) (First District)
Thomas A. Luken (Democrat) (Second District)
Tony P. Hall (Democrat) (Third District)
Michale Oxley (Republican) (Fourth District)
Delbert L. Latta (Republican) (Fifth District)
Bob McEwen (Republican) (Sixth District)
Clarence J. (Bud) Brown (Republican) (Seventh District)
Thomas N. Kindness (Republican) (Eighth District)
Ed Weber (Republican) (Ninth District)
Clarence E. Miller (Republican) (Tenth District)
J. William Stanton (Republican) (Eleventh District)
Robert N. (Bob) Shamansky (Democrat) (Twelfth District)
Donald J. (Don) Pease (Democrat) (Thirteenth District)
John F. Seiberling (Democrat) (Fourteenth District)
Chalmers P. Wylie (Republican) (Fifteenth District)
Ralph S. Regula (Republican) (Sixteenth District)
John M. Ashbrook (Republican) (Seventeenth District)
Douglas Applegate (Democrat) (Eighteenth District)
Lyle Williams (Republican) (Nineteenth District)
Mary Rose Oakar (Democrat) (Twentieth District)
Louis Stokes (Democrat) (Twenty-First District)
Dennis E. Eckart (Democrat) (Twenty-Second District)
Ronald M. Mottl (Democrat) (Twenty-Third District)

OKLAHOMA
Senate
David Lyle Boren (Democrat)
Don Nickles (Republican)
House of Representatives
James R. Jones (Democrat) (First District)
Michale Lynn (Mike) Synar (Democrat) (Second District)
Wes Watkins (Democrat) (Third District)
Dave McCurdy (Democrat) (Fourth District)
Mickey Edwards (Republican) (Fifth District)
Glenn English (Democrat) (Sixth District)

OREGON
Senate
Mark O. Hatfield (Republican)
Robert W. (Bob) Packwood (Republican)
House of Representatives
Les AuCoin (Democrat) (First District)
Denny Smith (Republican) (Second District)
Ron Wyden (Democrat) (Third District)
James (Jim) Weaver (Democrat) (Fourth District)

PENNSYLVANIA
Senate
H. John Heinz III (Republican)
Arlen Specter (Republican)
House of Representatives
Thomas M. Foglietta (Democrat) (First District)
William H. Gray III (Democrat) (Second District)
Joseph Smith (Democrat) (Third District)
Charles F. Dougherty (Republican) (Fourth District)
Richard T. Schulze (Republican) (Fifth District)
Gus Yatron (Democrat) (Sixth District)
Robert W. (Bob) Edgar (Democrat) (Seventh District)
James K. Coyne (Republican) (Eighth District)
E. G. (Bud) Shuster (Republican) (Ninth District)
Joseph M. McDade (Republican) (Tenth District)
James L. Nelligan (Republican) (Eleventh District)
John P. Murtha, Jr. (Democrat) (Twelfth District)
Lawrence Couglin (Republican) (Thirteenth District)
William J. Coyne (Democrat) (Fourteenth District)
Donald L. (Don) Ritter (Republican) (Fifteenth District)
Robert S. Walker (Republican) (Sixteenth District)
Allen E. Ertel (Democrat) (Seventeenth District)
Douglas (Doug) Walgren (Democrat) (Eighteenth District)
William F. (Bill) Goodling (Republican) (Nineteenth District)
Joseph M. Gaydos (Democrat) (Twentieth District)
Don Bailey (Democrat) (Twenty-First District)
Austin J. Murphy (Democrat) (Twenty-Second District)
William F. (Bill) Clinger, Jr. (Republican) (Twenty-Third District)
Marc Lincoln Marks (Republican) (Twenty-Fourth District)
Eugene V. Atkinson (Republican) (Twenty-Fifth District)

RHODE ISLAND
Senate
Claiborne Pell (Democrat)
John H. Chafee (Republican)
House of Representatives
Fernand J. St Germain (Democrat) (First District)
Claudine Schneider (Republican) (Second District)

SOUTH CAROLINA

Senate
Strom Thurmond (Republican)
Ernest F. Hollings (Democrat)
House of Representatives
Thomas F. Hartnett (Republican) (First District)
Floyd Spence (Republican) (Second District)
Butler Derrick (Democrat) (Third District)
Carroll A. Campbell, Jr. (Republican) (Fourth District)
Kenneth L. (Ken) Holland (Democrat) (Fifth District)
John L. Napier (Republican) (Sixth District)

SOUTH DAKOTA

Senate
Larry Pressler (Republican)
James Abdnor (Republican)
House of Representatives
Thomas A. Daschle (Democrat) (First District)
Clint Roberts (Republican)

TENNESSEE

Senate
Howard H. Baker, Jr. (Republican)
James R. Sasser (Democrat)
House of Representatives
James H. (Jimmy) Quillen (Republican) (First District)
John J. Duncan (Republican) (Second District)
Marilyn Lloyd Bouquard (Democrat) (Third District)
Albert Gore, Jr. (Democrat) (Fourth District)
William Hill (Bill) Boner (Democrat) (Fifth District)
Robin L. Beard, Jr. (Republican) (Sixth District)
Ed Jones (Democrat) (Seventh District)
Harold E. Ford (Democrat) (Eighth District)

TEXAS

Senate
John Tower (Republican)
Lloyd Bentsen (Democrat)
House of Representatives
Sam B. Hall, Jr. (Democrat) (First District)
Charles Wilson (Democrat) (Second District)
James M. (Jim) Collins (Republican) (Third District)
Ralph M. Hall (Democrat) (Fourth District)
Jim Mattox (Democrat) (Fifth District)
Phil Gramm (Democrat) (Sixth District)
Bill Archer (Republican) (Seventh District)
Jack Fields (Republican) (Eighth District)
Jack Brooks (Democrat) (Ninth District)
J. J. (Jake) Pickle (Democrat) (Tenth District)
J. Marvin Leath (Democrat) (Eleventh District)
Jim Wright (Democrat) (Twelfth District)

Jack Hightower (Democrat) (Thirteenth District)
William N. Patman (Democrat) (Fourteenth District)
E. (Kika) de la Garza (Democrat) (Fifteenth District)
Richard C. White (Democrat) (Sixteenth District)
Charles W. Stenholm (Democrat) (Seventeenth District)
Mickey Leland (Democrat) (Eighteenth District)
Kent Hance (Democrat) (Nineteenth District)
Henry B. Gonzalez (Democrat) (Twentieth District)
Thomas G. (Tom) Loeffler (Republican) (Twenty-First District)
Ron Paul (Republican) (Twenty-Second District)
Abraham Kazen, Jr. (Democrat) (Twenty-Third District)
Martin Frost (Democrat) (Twenty-Fourth District)

UTAH
Senate
Jacob (Jake) Garn (Republican)
Orrin G. Hatch (Republican)
House of Representatives
James V. Hansen (Republican) (First District)

VERMONT
Senate
Robert T. Stafford (Republican)
Patrick J. Leahy (Democrat)
House of Representatives
James M. Jeffords (Republican)

VIRGINIA
Senate
Harry F. Byrd, Jr. (Independent)
John W. Warner (Republican)
House of Representatives
Paul S. Trible, Jr. (Republican) (First District)
G. William Whitehurst (Republican) (Second District)
Thomas J. Bliley, Jr. (Republican) (Third District)
Robert W. Daniel, Jr. (Republican) (Fourth District)
W. C. (Dan) Daniel (Democrat) (Fifth District)
M. Caldwell Butler (Republican) (Sixth District)
J. Kenneth Robinson (Republican) (Seventh District)
Stanford E. Parris (Republican) (Eighth District)
William C. Wampler (Republican) (Ninth District)
Frank R. Wolf (Republican) (Tenth District)

WASHINGTON
Senate
Henry M. Jackson (Democrat)
Slade Gorton (Republican)
House of Representatives
Joel Pritchard (Republican) (First District)
Al Swift (Democrat) (Second District)
Don Bonker (Democrat) (Third District)

Sid Morrison (Republican) (Fourth District)
Thomas S. Foley (Democrat) (Fifth District)
Norman D. Dicks (Democrat) (Sixth District)
Michael E. (Mike) Lowry (Democrat) (Seventh District)

WEST VIRGINIA
Senate
Jennings Randolph (Democrat)
Robert C. Byrd (Democrat)
House of Representatives
Robert H. Mollohan (Democrat) (First District)
Cleveland K. Benedict (Republican) (Second District)
David Michael (Mick) Staton (Republican) (Third District)
Nick Joe Rahall II (Democrat) (Fourth District)

WISCONSIN
Senate
William Proxmire (Democrat)
Robert W. Kasten, Jr. (Republican)
House of Representatives
Les Aspin (Democrat) (First District)
Robert W. Kastenmeier (Democrat) (Second District)
Steven Gunderson (Republican) (Third District)
Clement J. Zablocki (Democrat) (Fourth District)
Henry S. Reuss (Democrat) (Fifth District)
Thomas E. Petri (Republican) (Sixth District)
David R. Obey (Democrat) (Seventh District)
Toby Roth (Republican) (Eighth District)
F. James Sensenbrenner, Jr. (Republican) (Ninth District)

WYOMING
Senate
Malcolm Wallop (Republican)
Alan K. Simpson (Republican)
House of Representatives
Richard Bruce (Dick) Cheney (Republican)

PUERTO RICO
Resident Commissioner
Baltasar Corrada (Democrat)

AMERICAN SAMOA
Delegate to Congress
Fofo I. F. Sunia (Independent)

DISTRICT OF COLUMBIA
Delegate to Congress
Walter E. Fauntroy (Democrat)

GUAM
Delegate to Congress
Antonio B. Won Pat (Democrat)

VIRGIN ISLANDS
Delegate to Congress
Ron de Lugo (Democrat)

TWO MORE IMPORTANT
BOOKS ON THE NUCLEAR ISSUE

☐ **NUCLEAR MADNESS by Dr. Helen Caldicott**
(#22774-2 · $3.50)

Nuclear technology threatens life on our planet with extinction. If present trends continue, the air we breathe, the food we eat, and the water we drink will soon be contaminated with enough radioactive pollutants to pose a potential health hazard far greater than any plague humanity has ever experienced. Dr. Helen Caldicott—pediatrician, mother of three and the President of Physicians for Social Responsibility—has written a concise, eloquent book which clearly describes the dangers of nuclear madness and tells you how you can make your voice heard.

☐ **HIROSHIMA by John Hersey (#20598-6 · $2.50)**

Absolutely essential reading for all people concerned about the threat of nuclear war. HIROSHIMA is John Hersey's classic masterpiece of what happened when the first atomic bomb was dropped thereby heralding a new era of nuclear war. Told through the experience of survivors, this is a timeless, powerful, compassionate document that has become a touchstone with lasting political and moral reverberations. "Nothing that can be said about this book can equal what the book has to say. It speaks for itself, and, in an unforgettable way, for humanity."—*The New York Times*